DESIGN, EXECUTION, AND MANAGEMENT OF MEDICAL DEVICE CLINICAL TRIALS

DESIGN, EXECUTION, AND MANAGEMENT OF MEDICAL DEVICE CLINICAL TRIALS

SALAH ABDEL-ALEEM

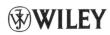

A JOHN WILEY & SONS, INC., PUBLICATION

For general information on our other products and services or for technical support, please
contact our Customer Care Department within the United States at (800) 762-2974, outside the
United States at (317) 572-3993 or fax (317) 572-4002.

Wiley also publishes its books in a variety of electronic formats. Some content that appears in
print may not be available in electronic formats. For more information about Wiley products,
visit our web site at www.wiley.com.

Library of Congress Cataloging-in-Publication Data:
Abdel-aleem, Salah.
    Design, execution, and management of medical device clinical trials / Salah Abdel-aleem.
        p. ; cm.
    Includes bibliographical references and index.
    ISBN 978-0-470-47426-6 (cloth)
    1. Medical instruments and apparatus–Research. 2. Clinical trials. I. Title.
    [DNLM: 1. Equipment and Supplies–standards. 2. Clinical Trials as Topic–methods.
3. Device Approval–standards. 4. Evaluation Studies as Topic.   W 26 A135d 2009]
    R856.4.A23 2009
    610.28′4—dc22
                                                                            2008049904

10 9 8 7 6 5 4 3 2 1

Dedication

For my mother, Farha, my loving wife, Maro, and my sons Omar, Tarek, and Yussuf. Your support has been truly inspirational.

CONTENTS

LIST OF ABBREVIATIONS

AE	Adverse event
ACE	Angiotensin converting enzyme
ANDA	Abbreviated new drug application
ARR	Absolute risk reduction
BMS	Bare metal stent
CBER	Center for Biologics Evaluation and Research (FDA)
CDHR	Center for Devices and Radiological Health (FDA)
CDER	Center for Drug Evaluation and Research (FDA)
CE marking	A mandatory European marking for certain product groups to indicate conformity with the essential health and safety requirements set out in European directives
CFR	Code of federal regulation
CMS	Centers for Medicare and Medicaid Services
CRA	Clinical research associate
CRFs	Case report forms
CRPAC	Clinical research policy analysis and coordination
CRO	Clinical research organization
CLI	Critical limb ischemia
DCFs	Data correction forms
DES	Drug eluting stent
DOB	Date of birth

DOD	Date of death
DSMB	Data safety monitoring board
EC	Ethics committee
ELA	Excimer laser atherectomy
FDA	Food and Drug Administration
FWA	Federal wide assurance
LACI	Laser angioplasty for critical limb ischemia
LOI	Letter of intent
GCP	Good clinical practice
GMDN	Global medical device nomenclature
HDE	Humanitarian device exemption
HIPAA	Health Insurance Portability Accountability Act
HUD	Humanitarian use device
ICF	Informed consent form
IDE	Investigational device exemption
IND	Investigational new drug
IRB	Institutional review board
NDA	New drug application
NIH	National Institute of Health
NSR	Nonsignificant risk
MACE	Major adverse cardiac events
MI	Myocardial infarction
OHRP	Office of Human Research Protection
OPC	Objective performance criteria
PAD	Peripheral artery disease
PI	Principal investigator
PMA	Premarket approval
PTA	Percutaneous transluminal angioplasty
RAS	Renin-angiotensin system
RRR	Relative risk reduction
SAE	Serious adverse event
SAP	Statistical analysis plan
SFA	Superficial femoral artery
SR	Significant risk
SOP	Standard operating procedures

SSN	Social security number
TASC	TransAtlantic Inter-Societal Consensus
TLR	Target lesion revascularization
TVR	Target vessel revascularization
UADE	Unanticipated adverse device effect
WHC	Weighted historic control

PREFACE

Clinical trial tasks and activities are widely diverse and require certain skill sets and educational backgrounds to both plan and execute. Among the various requirements needed for conducting clinical trials are management and communication skills, the ability to develop different clinical scientific and administrative documents (e.g., study protocols, case report forms, statistical analysis plans, final clinical reports, clinical standard operating procedures, and investigator brochures), and adequate monitoring experience. This book is designed to benefit people who work in the field of clinical research, specifically, although not limited to, clinical scientists, clinical managers, biostatisticians, clinical research associates, data management personnel, and clinical coordinators. Developed as a training manual, this book provides professionals with both an in-depth and broad range of knowledge of clinical research tasks and activities that will enable them to execute these tasks and activities successfully.

Specifically, this book provides a comprehensive review on the following topics:

- An overview of clinical trial tasks and activities starting with the preparation of clinical study materials and selection of clinical sites and ending with the completion of the final clinical study report
- A review of the FDA and ICH regulations applicable to medical devices

- A brief introduction of the use of biostatistics for sample size determination and study endpoints
- An outline and discussion of the final clinical study report
- Adverse event definitions, classifications, reporting, and analysis
- Challenging issues and obstacles in designing clinical studies
- Investigator-initiated clinical trials
- A review of clinical research bioethics

While this book is intended to serve as a training manual for professionals working with medical device clinical trials, several of these tasks are also applicable to drugs and biologics trials. Throughout this book practical examples compiled from previous clinical trial experiences are discussed in a sequential manner as they occurred in the study, starting from the development of the clinical protocol, progressing to selection of clinical sites, and ending with the completion of the final clinical report study.

After reading this book, the reader will be able to understand the function and responsibilities of each member of the clinical research team. In addition, the reader will acquire a comprehensive understanding of regulations, good clinical practices (GCP), and clinical standard operating procedures (SOP), which cover medical device clinical development and can be applied to everyday clinical operations for conducting and monitoring clinical trials. By nature, the subject material of this book is expansive. Certain topics, such as the international regulations of clinical trials, were considered beyond the scope of this project and are only briefly discussed. This book focuses on the FDA regulations of the United States. International regulations, although important, were considered to be outside the scope of this project. Notwithstanding, select references to international regulations, especially those in which the sponsor plans to include international sites as part of the FDA study, have been included. Finally, this book is not intended to discuss the statistical principals of clinical trial design in depth, but rather provide a simple approach in order to enable the reader to understand main terms, statistical procedures, sample size determination, study hypothesis, among other things.

The first four chapters of this book discuss clinical trial tasks and activities and instruct the reader how to perform these activities. This portion of the book provides an overview of tasks and definitions as well as instruction on managing and tracking the progress of these tasks. A presentation of the functions and responsibilities of every member of the clinical team is discussed in the first chapter to assist the reader to understand the integrative clinical tasks and activities required for the completion of a clinical study and how to manage these activities effectively. Chapter 2 discusses a manual of procedures on how to develop key documents required for clinical trials. Instructions and practical examples are given in this chapter on developing the clinical protocol, case report forms (CRF), clinical standard operating procedures (SOP), informed consent form (ICF), instructions for use (IFU), study regulatory binder, and other clinical forms required for the trial. The instructions for these documents include the thought process in developing the document, an outline of the content of each document, and actual examples of some of these documents such as CRF and clinical SOP. In this chapter, there is a discussion of methods and procedures used to ensure the quality and integrity of the data of a trial, such as selection of investigators, design of randomized blind study, the use of case report forms, institutional review board/ethical committee (IRB/EC), use of core laboratories, study committees, monitoring procedures/monitoring plan, defining protocol deviations, and defining study record retention and study reports. In continuation with the instructions for tasks and activities of clinical research, Chapter 3 provides a detailed discussion of the qualification and selection of study investigators and study sites. This chapter also includes discussions of the different types of study visits by the sponsor such as study initiation visit, interim monitoring visits, and study close out visits. The responsibilities of the study monitors are discussed in accordance with the type of site visit. At the end of this chapter, a presentation and examples of study monitoring reports are discussed.

The following chapters in the book, Chapters 4 through 6, are designed to cover the safety and effectiveness outcome of the study and statistical methods used to determine the outcome of the trial. In Chapter 4, a presentation of the definition of adverse events is discussed in accordance with the FDA and ICH guidelines. Chapter 4 is devoted to the definition of adverse events, serious adverse events, and unanticipated adverse device effects in accordance with the FDA and ICH guidelines. Also in this chapter, guidance is given to the investigator on the potential anticipated adverse events, what information needs to be reported about each adverse event, and the timeline for reporting different types of adverse events, as well as to whom they will report these adverse events. This chapter further defines what types of adverse events need be reported throughout the follow-up visits, after the completion of the research procedure. The analysis of adverse events as specified in the statistical analysis plan (SAP) is discussed. A definition is provided for what is considered a device-related adverse event, serious adverse event, unanticipated device adverse effect, and the grading of the severity or strength of adverse events. Chapter 5 provides a brief discussion of the statistical methods used in a clinical study and the statistical analysis plan (SAP). An outline and the contents of the SAP are discussed, followed by a brief discussion of statistical methods used in a clinical study, such as determination of the study sample size and power of a study. Instructions and recommendations are given in this chapter on how to eliminate or minimize the bias in a clinical trial. After reading this chapter, the reader will become familiar with simple statistic procedures and terms used for clinical studies. However, it should be noted that this chapter is not intended to provide detailed statistic analysis methods and procedures for clinical studies. Chapter 6 is devoted to discussing the final study clinical report. This activity is considered one of the most important activities in the clinical study, and enough time and resources should be assigned to complete this task because the FDA acceptance of a clinical study is largely dependent on this activity. This chapter starts with an outline of the final clinical report and then discusses each item in this outline. This chapter includes discussions of other important items in the report, such as missing data analysis, examination of data across study sites, and subgroup analysis.

Chapter 7 presents key FDA regulations applicable to medical devices, such as premarket notification using 510 (K), investigational device exempt (IDE), premarket application (PMA), and humanitarian device exemption (HDE). Regulations regarding combination products (e.g., drug eluting stent and drug delivery systems) are also reviewed in this chapter. Other FDA regulations have impact on the development of clinical tasks, and the chapter includes activities such as FDA-sponsor meetings (e.g., pre-IDE meetings), institutional review board (IRB) functions and responsibilities, special study committees (e.g., data safety monitoring board, clinical event adjudication, and steering committees), the HIPAA privacy rule, and bioresearch monitoring. It should be noted that this book is focused on the US medical device regulations of the FDA, and international regulations, although is important, are largely deemed beyond the scope of this book.

Chapter 8 reviews some challenging issues in designing clinical studies, such as the selection of historic control as the control group of the trial and the conduct of superiority versus noninferiority trial. This chapter also presents the data analysis of two PMA studies that used the historic control approach in its clinical studies. This chapter ends with recommendations for studies that use historic control and requirements of this control.

Chapter 9 provides a brief presentation of the investigator-sponsored clinical trials, particularly on the logistics of these studies. There is an increasing body of evidence that suggests an increased number of these trials, particularly in academic institutions funded by federal sources or private industry. Unlike clinical studies sponsored by biopharmaceutical or medical device companies, the sponsor of investigator-initiated research is usually an academic institution or private group of investigators. The sponsor of the study is usually responsible for the financial support, protocol development, product provision, conduct, and management of the study.

Chapter 10 presents the bioethics principles that were developed after World War II, such as the Declaration of Helsinki, and the Belmont Report. Special ethical concerns in clinical trials, such as regarding the use of placebo group in clinical research, are discussed as well.

A glossary of important clinical and statistical terms used in clinical research is presented in Chapter 11 of this book to get the reader familiar with the clinical and statistical terms used.

In summary, this book is intended to provide valuable information for clinical scientists (biostatisticians and clinical data analysis experts)—who develop and execute scientific clinical tasks, such as clinical protocols, statistical analysis plan (SAP), and final clinical protocol reports—as well as research associates—who manage and monitor clinical sites. Additionally, this book is a valuable resource for clinical managers needing to develop an integrative vision of all clinical research activities in order to plan and execute clinical studies effectively.

SALAH ABDEL-ALEEM, PhD

Senior Clinical Operation Manager
Proteus Biomedical, Inc.

To view supplemental material for this book, please visit ftp://ftp.wiley.com/public/sci_tech_med/design_execution.

ACKNOWLEDGMENTS

I would not have the opportunity to write this book without having collaborated with the following wonderful professors and mentors: Professor M. El-Merzabani at the Egyptian National Cancer Institute, who taught me the principles of laboratory research after graduating from college; Professor Horst Schulz of the City University of New York, my PhD supervisor; Professor James E. Lowe at the Duke University Medical Center, who I collaborated with for eight years in cardiac research; Professors Daniel Burkhoff and William Gray at Columbia University, who provided me with invaluable insight on clinical studies; Dr. Mohamed Nada, friend and colleague; Professor Ismail Sallam, the former Egyptian Minister of Health; and my colleagues at Proteus Biomedical Inc., particularly Dr. Greg Moon, Dr. George Savage, and Dr. Allison Intondi. Last, but not least, my students and those who I have mentored. These individuals helped shape my scientific career and motivated me to write this book.

1

AN OVERVIEW OF CLINICAL STUDY TASKS AND ACTIVITIES

Design, Execution, and Management of Medical Device Clinical Trials,
by Salah Abdel-aleem
Copyright © 2009 John Wiley & Sons, Inc.

KEY CLINICAL STUDY TASKS AND ACTIVITIES

This chapter provides an overview of the clinical tasks and activities that are required for planning and executing clinical studies. Usually all of the clinical activities are completed in a pivotal clinical study (an adequate size confirmatory study to demonstrate the safety and effectiveness of the investigational product); however, in some observatory clinical trials some of these steps may be reduced or eliminated altogether. The diversity and complexity of these tasks may require a clinical team that consists of people of certain skill sets (e.g., clinical managers, clinical scientists, biostatisticians, data management personnel, and clinical research associates) in order to complete these activities successfully. This chapter presents an overview of the key clinical deliverables (the details of each sub-activity task are discussed in the following chapters), such as, the development of the clinical protocol includes other sub-activity tasks, such as the development of the protocol synopsis, detailed study procedures, statistical section, administrative section, and finally the entire protocol. The clinical tasks and activities are arranged in this chapter in a sequential manner as they occur in the clinical study, starting with the development of the study clinical protocol and ending with the completion of the final clinical report. In this introductory chapter, methods of management of the clinical tasks by study managers are presented. In addition a presentation of the different members of the clinical team and their role and responsibilities is discussed in this chapter. In summary, this chapter will help the reader to keep an integrative view of all key tasks and activities required for a clinical studies and how to manage these activities effectively. At the end of this chapter the reader should get familiar with all clinical tasks as well as the order of these tasks required for a clinical study.

The following is a *list of the key clinical deliverables for a clinical study*:

1. Development of the clinical protocol and study materials
2. Qualification and selection of the clinical investigators and study sites
3. FDA approval for the study if required
4. IRB approval of the protocol, informed consent form (ICF), and advertising materials
5. Study research contract
6. Study initiation visit

7. First patient in (first patient enrollment)
8. Last patient out (last patient completed last follow-up visit)
9. Study close-out
10. Database lock (all data for the study are entered into the database)
11. Generation of data queries
12. Database cleaning
13. Development of the final study clinical report
14. Study progress reports

DISCUSSION OF KEY TASKS AND ACTIVITIES

Development of the Clinical Protocol and Study Materials

Development of the clinical protocol is one of the earliest activities in a clinical study. The clinical protocol considered one of the most important documents for the study, as it describes the background, purpose, objectives, design, and procedures for the study. Enough time and resources should be given to the process of developing the clinical protocol. Each section in the protocol should be clearly written to avoid confusion and misinterpretation. The protocol is also a dynamic document in the sense that it can be revised or amended, even after starting the study, if there is a need to clarify or modify certain procedures.

The development of the clinical protocol may require effort from several clinical research staff members working at or for the sponsor of the study and may also require input from leading clinical researchers in each area of research. Clinical experts and key researchers can provide valuable information on the proposed patient population, study endpoints, and its measurements, and the experimental procedures of the trial. Once the clinical protocol is established, templates for other clinical materials, such as the case report form and the informed consent form template, are developed in accordance with it.

The creation of protocol synopsis (protocol summary) is the first step in developing the clinical protocol. This document is usually a few pages long and includes the study title, purpose, patient selection criteria (inclusion or exclusion criteria), endpoints, and experimental procedures. This document can be used in the early preparation phase of the trial to communicate the proposed study with the potential clinical investigators.

The following study details should be clearly explained and discussed in the clinical protocol:

- Basis for sample size calculation and anticipated power of the study
- How patients are recruited and randomized to groups (this is illustrated in patients enrollment flowchart)
- Define patient selection criteria (this is defined by setting up specific inclusion/exclusion criteria)
- Methods of blinding
- Planned subgroups and interim analysis
- Study special committees (e.g., Data Safety Monitoring Board, Clinical Event Adjudication Committee, and Steering Committee)
- Data quality assurance procedures

For more on the process of development of the clinical protocol, see Chapter 2: "The Development of the Clinical Protocol, Case Report Forms, Clinical Standard Operating Procedures, Informed Consent Form, Regulatory Study Binder, and Other Clinical Materials."

Qualification and Selection of Investigators and Clinical Sites

Potential clinical investigators and clinical sites should be carefully selected in the preparation for the study. The selection of the principal investigator (PI) and study sites is discussed in Chapter 3. The process of qualifying and selecting investigators and clinical sites can be summarized as follows:

- To ensure the confidentiality of the product and study information, a Confidentiality Agreement is usually signed by the potential investigator prior to exchanging information about the study or the study product.
- The study sponsor representative contacts the potential investigators and sends out the protocol synopsis to find out if they are interested in participating in the study.
- The sponsor may schedule a qualification visit to further evaluate interested investigators and their clinical sites for adequacy for the proposed trial.
- After the final selection process is completed, a letter is sent out to these investigators informing them whether or not they were selected for the study.

FDA Approval for the Study (If Required)

If the product is determined to present significant risk and the study is conducted under, for example, an IDE (Investigationanl Device Exemption), the sponsor must obtain FDA approval for the study prior to conducting the research. This may also require early discussion with the FDA about the proposed study to ensure that the FDA finds it acceptable. The discussion between the FDA and the sponsor usually focuses in the selection of the patient population, the indication for the treatment, study endpoints, and study procedures. Communication between the FDA and the sponsor is initiated by the sponsor requesting a pre-IDE meeting with the FDA. For more details on this process, see section under FDA-Sponsor Meetings in Chapter 7. Additionally the sponsor may want to invite clinical experts to participate in this meeting if their participation is essential in highlighting certain clinical issues pertaining to the proposed study to the FDA. Early communication between the study sponsor and the FDA is highly encouraged to prevent any confusion about the planned study between the sponsor and the FDA. The sponsor should feel confident that the FDA agrees with the proposed study design (patient population, indication, study endpoints, and study procedures).

Institutional Review Board/Ethics Committee (IRB/EC) Approval of the Protocol, the Informed Consent Form (ICF), and the Study of Advertising Materials

IRB/EC must approve the study protocol, informed consent form, and study advertising materials. If the study is conducted under the IDE process, a majority of the reviewing IRBs require the FDA approval prior to their review and approval. A summaries of the role and responsibility of the IRB are presented in Chapters 2 and 7. Certain clinical sites use local IRB; other sites use central IRB. Enough time should be given to get the IRB approval, particularly in sites that use local IRB. The preparation of the study and the approval of the local IRB could take two to three months. The central IRB approval is usually obtained in less time.

Study Research Contract

A signed research contract between the sponsor and the study site or research investigator must be completed prior to initiating the study. Enough time should be given to complete this activity especially when dealing with academic sites, which tend to take longer time than private clinical sites.

The research contract includes the following points:

- The name, title, and address of the parties involved
- Responsibilities of the principal investigator (PI)
- Subject injury reimbursement
- Payments to the clinical sites and the terms of payment
- Schedule of payments
- Deliverables required for payments
- Indemnification
- Publication policy

The research contract is a legally binding agreement involving four main points:

- Offer: From pharmaceutical/medical device company as the sponsor
- Acceptance: By institution and investigator
- For services and results: By institution and investigator
- In exchange for money: From sponsor to conduct the research/trial

The structure and template of the research contracted are presented in Chapter 2.

Study Initiation Visit

The sponsor conducting the study initiates a visit to train the principal investigator and the research team at the clinical site on the protocol, the investigational product, study procedures, and good clinical practice (GCP) issues, including the responsibilities of the principal investigator and research team in the reporting of adverse events, and obtaining consent of study subjects. This visit is typically conducted following FDA and IRB approval for the study, and the investigational product is received at the site. It is preferred that the visit be scheduled as close as possible to the enrollment of the first subject in the trial. During this training the sponsor should use various presentation and device models to describe and give details of the study. The sponsor representative(s) conducting this visit should file the name and title of every attendee of this training in the study training log. In certain studies the sponsor may want to administer a quiz at the end of this visit to ensure an adequate level of understanding of the study by the attendees of the training (see Chapter 3 for more details on the study initiation visit).

First Patient In

This term means that the first patient is enrolled in the study after the subject met all study eligibility criteria. This is considered a key milestone in the clinical trial because it marks the actual initiation of patient enrollment in the study.

It is important to define in the study protocol the exact meaning of the phrase "enrolled subject or patient in the trial." Does it means subjects who have met all eligibility criteria and have completed all baseline assessments, or does it refer to randomized subjects? Does it entail whether the investigational device has been implanted or will be implanted in the study subjects?

Last Patient Out

This term implies that last subject enrolled in the study has completed all study follow-up visits in accordance with the study protocol. Study follow-up visits range from several weeks or months (short term follow-up visits) to one year or longer (long-term follow-up visits). This event is also considered an important milestone in a clinical study because it designates the end of patient follows-up visits in the clinical trial.

Study Close-Out

The study close-out visit is completed once all subjects complete the follow-up visits, and once investigational device inventories are completed and copies of all CRFs are retrieved. For more details on this topic, see Chapter 3.

Database Lock

This term is used by data management personnel to indicate that all data for the study have been entered into the database and no additional patient data will be entered into the database after this date except data pertaining to the cleaning of the existing database. However, it should be noted that there are a few exceptions to the rule. For example, new significant data available to the study as well as long-term follow-up data can be entered into the database after it has been locked.

Generation of Data Queries

All data queries for data inconsistency for the study that is entered into the database are generated on data correction forms (DCFs) or other forms and sent out to clinical study sites for clarification and correction. The study sites correct and clarify these data inconsistencies in the designated DCFs or CRFs, and send this information back to the sponsor. Copies of the corrected DCFs will be kept in patient clinical study files at the study sites and the sponsor files.

Database Cleaning

This process is conducted after receiving DCFs, or corrected CRFs from the study sites that contained data inconsistency, to clean up the data in the database. After the database cleaning the final data of the study are generated in form of various tables, charts, and figures in accordance with the statistical analysis plan (SAP).

Development of the Final Study Clinical Report

This represents the final task in the clinical study. The development of the final clinical report is a task that requires the input of several members on the clinical research team. The final study clinical report writing team typically consists of a report writing person, a biostatistician, and the clinical experts who have analyzed the clinical data. The final clinical report contains several sections, including a section on special procedures followed in the study to ensure the quality of the trial, analysis and discussion of patient baseline characteristics, study endpoints, and analysis of adverse events (for more detail on the content of this report, see Chapter 6).

Study Progress Reports

At least once a year the sponsor must provide reports to all reviewing IRB. For significant risk devices, the sponsor must also submit the progress report to the FDA.

A Template of an Outline of the FDA Annual Progress Report   An outline of the FDA annual progress report should include the following items:

1. *Basic Elements*
   - IDE number

- Device name and indication(s) for use
- Sponsor's name, address, phone number, and fax
- Contact person

2. Study Progress
   - Brief summary of the study progress in relation to the investigational plan
   - Number of investigators/investigational sites (attach list of investigators)
   - Number of subjects enrolled (by indication or model)
   - Number of devices shipped
   - Brief summary of results
   - Summary of anticipated and unanticipated adverse effects
   - Description of any deviations from the investigational plan by investigators (since last progress report)

3. Risk Analysis
   - Summary of any new adverse information (since the last progress report) that may affect the risk analysis, such as preclinical data, animal studies, foreign data, and clinical studies
   - Reprints of any articles published from data collected from this study
   - New risk analysis, if necessary, based on new information and on study progress

4. Other Changes
   - Summary of any changes in manufacturing practices and quality control (e.g., changes not reported in a supplemental application)
   - Summary of all changes in the investigational plan not required to be submitted in a supplemental application

5. Future Plans
   - Progress toward product approval, with projected date of PMA or 510(k) submission
   - Any plans to change the investigation, such as to expand the study size or indications, to discontinue portions of the investigation, or to change manufacturing practices.

MANAGEMENT OF KEY CLINICAL TASKS AND ACTIVITIES

The project manager of the clinical study should use several tools to manage activities and track the progress of the tasks in the clinical study (Microsoft Excel spread sheets, Microsoft Manager, etc.). The management of these studies includes tracking the progress of the project activities (project timeline), managing the human resources available for the project, and managing the study budget (payments for sites, CRO, consultants, materials, etc.).

Documents that are used to track the progress of these activities should include a description of each activity, a planned completion date, the actual completion date, and a comment section to show whether an activity is controlled by any other activity and/or to discuss why the completion of a particular activity has been delayed from its anticipated date. For example, selecting the PI and clinical sites for a study may require that the sponsor be able to share information about the proposed clinical study to potential clinical sites. This may necessitate signing a confidentiality agreement document by the PI in order to share confidential information with the investigator, and the development of the protocol synopsis (i.e., the protocol summary) to survey the level of interest of the investigator prior to the selection of the investigators and study sites. In addition certain activities should pass through several phases (e.g., the qualification and selection of the investigators, which starts with the evaluation of the potential investigators and ends with the final selection of those investigators).

EXAMPLE OF THE SPREAD SHEET FOR MANAGING CLINICAL STUDY ACTIVITIES

It is helpful to track the progress of the key clinical deliverables in spread sheet. It should be noted that some of these activities are tracked in different phases. For example, approval of a study may demand several rounds between the FDA or IRB and the sponsor. This process could start by giving the sponsor a conditional approval and end several months later with a final approval after the sponsor clarifies certain issues in the study. Therefore the tracking process should be set up to take into account all of the different phases of the activity (approval of the study protocol, approval of protocol amendments, etc.).

Tracking of items should include the planned date of activity, the actual completion date, and a comment section on each activity to list the reasons why particular activity has been delayed (see table 1.1).

THE CLINICAL RESEARCH TEAM

The clinical research team at, or representing, the sponsor consists of the following members:

TABLE 1.1 Tracking of the Key Clinical Research Tasks and Activities

Activity/Task	Planned Date	Completion Data	Comments

Protocol development
  Protocol synopsis
  ICF template
  CRFs			

Qualification of potential sites Final selection of study sites			

FDA approval for the study
  Pre-IDE meeting
  Final FDA approval			

IRB approval for the study
  IRB submission
  Final IRB approval			

Study contract sign off			
Investigational device shipment			
Study initiation visit			
First patient in			
Last patient out			
Close-out visit			
All study CRFs in house			
Database Lock			
Study queries generation			
Study queries out to clinical sites			
Response to queries received			
Database cleaning			
Development of the final clinical report			
Development of the annual progress report			

Clinical Study Manager

This person is responsible for the following clinical tasks:

- Plan, manage, and execute clinical studies
- Plan the study timeline, budget, and resources
- Manage the development of the clinical protocol, ICF, CRFs, and other clinical materials
- Supervise and mentor study monitors

- Review monitoring reports
- Review the study adverse event reports
- Review clinical data

Clinical Research Associates (CRAs)

These personnel are responsible for the execution of the various activities in the study:

- Study setup and manage communications with clinical sites
- Prepare and execute of investigator meeting
- Conduct various study monitoring activities
- Write monitoring reports
- Review source documents for adverse events

Data Management Personnel

These personnel are responsible for managing the data of the study:

- Enter clinical study data into the study database
- Generate study tables and figures in accordance with the SAP and study protocol

Biostatistician

This person has the following responsibilities:

- Develop the Statistical Analysis Plan (SAP)
- Develop the statistics associated with the study's endpoints and determine the sample size assumptions
- Participate in the development of the final clinical reports
- Ensure that the protocol and any amendments cover all relevant statistical issues clearly and accurately
- Review the CRFs to ensure that primary and secondary endpoints are collected and/or captured appropriately to satisfy analyses called for in the SAP, where applicable
- Work with clinical data manager to update study plan if the SAP changes and if those changes reflect changes to data collected during the conduct of the clinical research trial

IRB Coordinator

This person is responsible for the following activities:

- Coordinate IRB submissions
- Serve as contact person for communications
- Write responses to IRB

Regulatory Specialist

This person has the following activities:

- Review clinical protocols, ICF, and other clinical materials to ensure that these documents were developed in accordance with applicable regulations
- Coordinate FDA pre-IDE meeting
- Serve as a liaison between the sponsor and FDA
- Responsible for communicating responses to FDA questions regarding any particular submission to the FDA

2

DEVELOPMENT OF CLINICAL PROTOCOLS, CASE REPORT FORMS, CLINICAL STANDARD OPERATING PROCEDURES, INFORMED CONSENT FORM, STUDY REGULATORY BINDER, STUDY RESEARCH AGREEMENT, AND OTHER CLINICAL MATERIALS

Design, Execution, and Management of Medical Device Clinical Trials,
by Salah Abdel-aleem
Copyright © 2009 John Wiley & Sons, Inc.

The preparation of a clinical trial requires the development of several documents, clinical protocol, case report forms (CRFs), informed consent form (ICF), study regulatory binder, and other clinical materials that describe, control, and manage all aspects of the study. These documents are generally developed by the clinical scientists and clinical research associates at the sponsor. Additionally the clinical team may develop other documents, such as, clinical standard operating procedures (SOPs), that may already exist or are specially designed to provide guidelines for certain clinical practices. This chapter discusses in detail the development and the contents of all required study documents in accordance with all applicable regulations. Instructions are provided on how to develop these activities. Examples are given of outlines or contents of these documents (clinical protocol, case report forms, clinical standard operating procedures, etc.), and the items included in these documents are discussed. This chapter is one of the key instructional chapters in the book on how to develop the documents required for a clinical trial. The activity of development of a particular document goes through a process that involves the following steps: a thought process for planning the activity, an outline of the planned activity, details on outlined items, and practical examples of the final activity. For example, the development of the clinical a protocol goes through the following process: the preparing of a protocol synopsis (summary), the review of the protocol synopsis by clinical experts, development of the entire protocol, and review of the entire protocol by clinical and regulatory experts.

CLINICAL PROTOCOL

The clinical protocol contains purpose, intended use of the investigational therapy, patient population selection criteria, study endpoints and objectives of the research, study experimental procedures, and subjects' follow-up visits for the proposed trial. In addition this document includes other sections such as adverse event definitions and reporting, sample size determination and statistical methods, and procedures followed to ensure quality and integrity of the study data.

Protocol Development Process[1,2]

Protocol development is a process that requires the input from various members of the clinical research team (clinical experts, regulatory specialists, and biostatisticians). The research team typically assigns a qualified clinical research staff member to coordinate the development of the study protocol. The protocol development process include the following steps: (1) development of protocol synopsis by the sponsor, (2) review of the protocol synopsis by clinical experts and key thought leaders in this area of research, (3) development of the protocol draft, (4) review of the protocol draft by clinical and regulatory experts, and (5) development of the final protocol.

A protocol synopsis (summary) is initially prepared. It consists of few pages long and contains title, purpose of the study, indication for use, patient selection criteria, study endpoints/objectives, study experimental procedures, and follow-up visits. This document is discussed with a few clinical experts and clinical thought leaders in this area of research, to tune up the selection of the patient population, study endpoints, and study procedures. After the protocol synopsis is approved, the process of developing a draft of the entire protocol is initiated. The protocol draft will have more sections than what is already written in the protocol synopsis, such as sample size calculation and statistical analysis, adverse events definition and reporting, risk/benefit analysis, and methods used to ensure the quality and integrity of the study data. The draft of the final protocol should be reviewed again by the clinical and regulatory experts, especially the newly added sections, and then the final protocol is completed.

In global clinical studies, because international sites are planned to be included in the study and the final clinical report is probably going to be submitted to the FDA as well as other international regulatory bodies, early communications are encouraged with the US and the international clinical teams to make the regulations and procedures of the study protocol compatible with both foreign and US regulations. For example, correlations could be made in reporting units of measurements in the CRFs, adverse events, and the use of concomitant medications. Differences may exist between the US and other international sites in the reporting time periods of serious adverse events from the investigator to a the sponsor or to a regulatory authority. Also, to avoid confusion about the units of measurements between the US and international sites, alternatives for unit definitions should be provided, or clinical sites should be instructed on which units they should use in the study. Another area of concern is synchronization of the clinical protocol procedures in global clinical trials on the use of protocol concomitant medications. For economic or other reasons certain international sites use other, alternative, drugs than those used in the United States. To avoid having numerous protocol deviations, these alternative medications should be recognized in the study protocol if there is no effect on the study outcome (for more detail on the global clinical studies, see Chapter 8).

Development of the Clinical Protocol

The Research Question (Research Hypothesis)   The process of developing the clinical protocol starts by recognizing *the research question* (study question). The components of formulating a research hypothesis are as follow:

- *What is the study outcome?*   This is to be determined by variable selection and measurements.
- *What is the intervention?*   This needs a clear definition of the intervention.
- *When and for how long to treat?*   This is determined by the study design.
- *For whom treatment is designed?*   This determined by eligibility criteria.
- *What is the number of participants?*   This is determined by the sample size estimates.

• *How can the potential benefits be optimized and potential risks minimized?* This is managed by variable selection and measurements, eligibility criteria, and monitoring for safety and benefits.

An Outline of the Clinical Protocol   The clinical protocol includes the following sections:

1. Administrative Information
   a. Protocol title, protocol number, and version date. Any protocol amendments should also include the amendment number and date
   b. Name and address of the sponsor and monitor (if other than the sponsor)
   c. Name, title, address, and telephone number of the medical expert for the trial
2. Background and Rationale for the Study
   a. Background
      i. Description of the population to be studied
      ii. Summary of condition or disease to be treated including the economic impact of this condition
      iii. Summary of alternative treatments
      iv. Summary of potential risks and benefits to subjects
      v. Rational for the undertaken study
   b. Report of prior published and unpublished pre-clinical and clinical studies
   c. Device description
3. Purpose of the Study
4. Intended Use
5. Study Design
   a. Study overview
   b. Patients selection criteria
      i. Inclusion criteria
      ii. Exclusion criteria
   c. Study experimental procedures
   d. Study visits and follow-up visits
   e. Study endpoints or goals
      i. Primary endpoints
         1. Primary safety endpoint(s)

       2. Primary effectiveness or performance endpoint(s)

     ii. Secondary endpoints

     iii. Other endpoints

6. Sample Size Determination and Statistical Analysis
7. Adverse Events
    a. Definitions of adverse events
    b. Potential (anticipated) adverse events
    c. Adverse event reporting
        i. Description of adverse events
        ii. Serious adverse events
        iii. Unanticipated adverse device effects
        iv. Adverse event severity/strength
        v. Relatedness of adverse events to study product or study procedures
        vi. Serious adverse event narratives
    d. Time periods for adverse events reporting
8. Risk/Benefit Analysis
    a. Risks associated with the disease to be treated
    b. Risks associated with the study procedures
    c. Risks associated with the study device
    d. Mitigations of Risks
    e. Risk/benefit analysis
    f. Conclusion
9. Quality Assurance and Management of Data Collection
    a. Selection of Investigators
    b. Institutional review board/ethics committee
    c. Selection of core labs
    d. Case report forms
    e. Monitoring plan
    f. Study committees
    g. Protocol deviations
    h. Record retention
    i. Study reports
10. References
11. Attachments
    a. ICF
    b. Research contract template

Discussion of the Clinical Protocol Sections

Background and Rationale   The sponsor should identify the research criteria and source of collected literature for the study, such as the use of peer-reviewed journals, review articles, meta-analysis studies (including criteria used to select these studies). The background section should set up the stage for the proposed study with a clear rational for the need of the investigational therapy.

The background and rationale section includes the following:

- A review of literature about the disease or condition to be treated
- Frequency of the disease and economic impact of disease or condition
- Other available alternative therapies
- The rational for the proposed study
- Prior published and unpublished preclinical and clinical studies performed with the investigational product
- Description of the investigational device.

Purpose of the Study   A clear purpose for the study should be stated in the protocol. This statement should specify the purpose in terms of the following criteria:

- The patient population
- The projected clinical outcome

For example, the purpose of the study could be stated as follows: "This study is designed to evaluate the safety and effectiveness of XYZ device in the reduction of myocardial infarction in patients with coronary artery disease." It is clear from the purpose statement that the patient population is defined as patients with coronary artery disease and the clinical outcome of the study is defined as reduction of the myocardial infarction. The purpose of a feasibility study is stated little differently from that of a pivotal study. As in the previous example, the purpose of feasibility study could be worded as: "This study is designed to evaluate the initial safety and the feasibility of the performance of the XYZ device in patients with coronary artery disease."

Intended Use   The intended use of the device should characterize the precise patient population and define the clinical outcome of the study.

The intended use for the investigational therapy should be carefully worded to relate the study's outcome to selected patient population. In other words, the intended use should clearly state what the sponsor is going to claim for the investigational product.

Study Design   This section includes an overview of the study design. It indicates whether the study is randomized or nonrandomized, single or multicenter, open label, blinded or double-blinded, the number of subjects enrolled, and the expected duration of subject participation in the study. This section includes the maintenance of randomization codes and any procedures for breaking such codes if necessary. Additionally the study design section presents, step by step, the study experimental procedures (at baseline, during the procedure, after the completion of the procedure, and during study follow-up visits).

Study Endpoints   This section describes the primary, secondary, and other endpoints in the study. A clear definition of endpoints includes its measurements and a description of the study success parameters along with a determination of the significance level. The primary effectiveness endpoint(s) of the study should be specified with inclusion of methods and timing for assessing, recording, and analyzing parameters. Similarly secondary and other endpoints in the study should be defined with methods of measuring these endpoints (for detailed discussion on the study endpoints, see Chapter 5).

Eligibility Criteria   Eligibility criteria for the study are determined by specific inclusion and exclusion criteria that define precisely the patient population of the trial. The criteria should be:

- Stated in advance
- Selected to maximize potential effect of the intervention and minimize risks in selected population

The following issues should be carefully addressed by the sponsor when developing eligibility criteria for the study:

1. The precise eligibility criteria collected. For example, if the protocol requires the participation of nonpregnant female in the study, then:
   i. This criterion should be checked in the case report forms of the study, as nonapplicable, for potential male candidates.

    ii. Women of childbearing potential may not be routinely excluded from participating in research (unless they have positive pregnancy test); however, pregnant women should be excluded unless there is clear justification why they should be included.

2. Participation of adult subjects in research not age-restricted if there is no scientific or medical justification
3. Additional restrictions that may apply to minors or any other category of vulnerable subjects
4. Justification for any enrollment restrictions
5. Withdrawal criteria and procedures:
    i. When and how to withdraw subjects from the trial
    ii. Type and timing of data to be collected for withdrawn subjects
    iii. Whether and how drop out, or withdraw subjects are to be replaced
    iv. Follow-up for subjects that withdrawn from the trial and/or from using the experimental product

Study Experimental Procedures

It is helpful to summarize the protocol experimental procedures during screening/baseline assessments, during procedures, and follow-up visits in a table. The table should show the schedule of all protocol procedures and assessments as they occur in the study. An example is provided in Table 2.1.

The follow-up periods listed in the table are divided in accordance with the study follow-up visits of, for example, 1 month, 6 months, 12

TABLE 2.1   Schedule of Assessments in the Clinical Protocol

Assessment/Evaluation	Assessment Time Period			
	Screening	Baseline	Procedure	Follow Up Periods
Inclusion/exclusion criteria	X			
Pregnancy test	X			
Medical history		X		
Concomitant medications		X		
Physical exam		X		
Lab tests			X	
Imaging tests			X	
Adverse events			X	X

months, or more. When designing this activity (the schedule of assessments), it is also important to list all study physiological, laboratory, or life quality measurements used throughout the study.

Adverse events are reported from the time of patient or subject enrollment until the completion of the study follow-up period. However, in some studies certain serious or major adverse events are only reported during the follow-up period.

Sample Size Determination and Statistical Analysis   This section includes the following:

- Sample size assumptions
- The primary hypothesis of the study
- How proposed sample size is designed to prove the primary endpoint of the study
- Statistical method(s) used to analyze study endpoints including the level of significance to be used
- Criteria for terminating the study should be also described if there is a considerable safety concern
- Procedures for missing and unused data and procedures for reporting deviations from the original statistical plan should be described

To avoid a compromise in the power of the sample size after the study's completion, because of patients who are lost to follow-up, withdraw consent, or missed the primary endpoint assessments, it is recommended that the predetermined sample size of the study should include additional subjects than the calculated (e.g., 5% or 10% more subjects than the precalculated sample size). For more details on the sample size, determination, and statistical analysis, see Chapter 5.

Adverse Events   This section is discussed in detail in Chapter 4. Covered in this section are:

- Definitions of adverse events (adverse events, serious adverse events, and unanticipated adverse device effects)
- List of potential anticipated adverse events that may occur in the study
- Adverse event outcome (e.g., resolved, ongoing, resolved with residual damage)
- Adverse event severity or strength (e.g., mild, moderate, severe)

- Adverse event relationship to study device or study procedures (e.g., related, unrelated, unknown)
- Narratives of serious and major adverse events
- Time periods for reporting adverse events
- Methods of monitoring, reporting, and analyzing of adverse events

Risk/Benefit Analysis This section includes a discussion of risks associated with the disease to be treated, the theoretical risks and the reasonably foreseeable risks, and risk/benefit assessments for the investigational therapy. Separation should be made between theoretical risks and reasonably foreseeable risks. By analyzing the risks/benefits associated with the investigational product, the reviewer should get a clear sense of the benefits that a subject could have from participating in the study. Sometimes there is no direct benefit for the subject in participating in the study other than enhancing our knowledge about the disease process, diagnosis, or treatment that could be beneficial in future studies.

The risk/benefit analysis could be in the clinical protocol or in the investigational plan as a part of the IDE. After analyzing the risks/benefits of a new therapy, the reviewer should be able to conclude that the benefits of this therapy outweigh the potential risks for participating subjects. In summary, the risk/benefit analysis of a clinical study should include a discussion of the following issues:

- Risks associated with the disease to be treated
- Risks associated with the study procedures
- Risks associated with the study device
- Mitigations of risks
- Risks compared with benefits
- Summary of results

Study Quality Assurance and Management of Data Collection The following are examples of methods and procedures used to ensure the quality and integrity of the trial and collected data:

- Qualification and selection of investigator and clinical sites
- Randomization of study groups
- Blinding of subjects, treating physicians, and data analysis group
- Case report forms
- Institutional review board/ethics committee

- Core laboratories
- Study committees
- Monitoring procedures and monitoring plan
- Defining protocol deviations
- Defining record retention and study reports

Methods and Procedures Used to Ensure Quality and Integrity of the Trial

Selection of Investigators   A discussion should be included on how investigators and clinical sites are to be qualified and selected for the study. The criteria used for the selection process should be defined, such as that selection is based on investigator knowledge, experience, integrity, and ability to recruit required patient population in the proposed enrollment period. For more detail on this process, see Chapter 3.

Randomization and Blindness   The study clinical protocol for pivotal clinical studies should be designed as a randomized, blind study whenever is possible. It has been suggested that randomization and blindness play a key role in ensuring the quality of the trial. For more detail on randomization and blindness, see Chapter 8.

Study Case Report Forms (CRFs)   CRFs are designed to capture the data as described in the clinical protocol (demographic data, study outcome/measurements, adverse events, etc.). The sponsor should also provide to the study sites clear instructions on how to complete the CRFs. CRFs are monitored to ensure accuracy of reported data in accordance with source documents of the data. For more detail on CRFs, see section under "Case Report Forms" in this chapter.

IRB/Ethics Committees   This section explains the obligations and responsibilities of investigators toward their own reviewing IRB. Additionally the role of the IRBs/ECs is discussed in this section. A discussion of the roles and responsibilities of the reviewing IRB/EC: 21 CFR Part 56 covers the regulations of the IRB: IRB membership, IRB functions and operations, and so forth. The IRB responsibilities can be summarized as follow:

- Assures compliance with the federal wide assurance (FWA)
- Assures policies and procedures are effectively applied in compliance with state and federal laws and regulations

- Provides interpretation and application of federal regulations
- Develops, implements, and interprets IRB policies and procedures
- Takes action on noncompliance according to IRB policies and procedures, as necessary
- Performs and documents quality assurance activities to assure compliance
- Provides internal and external monitoring, which is designed to assess compliance and safety in human subjects research
- Performs directed audits and random compliance reviews; formulates and implements, as needed, recommendations for the Investigator and his/her staff

For more detail on the functions and responsibilities of the IRB, see Chapter 7.

Selection of Core Laboratories for the Study   The selection of core laboratories to function as central labs for the study should minimize or eliminate risks associated with the different interpretations of the test reports, since a single core lab will be responsible for interpreting and completing the reports in the study.

Monitoring Procedures and Monitoring Plan   This includes the frequency and type of monitoring visits, and what exactly the sponsor's representative will monitor in each monitoring visit. For more detail on this process, see Chapter 3.

Study Committees   Study committees, such as Data Safety Monitoring Board Committee (DSMB), Clinical Event Adjudication Committees (CEC), and Steering Committee, are set up to achieve the following objectives:

- Review and ensure patients safety data
- Provide uniform definitions and criteria to identify serious or major adverse events
- Recommend stopping the study if serious concern arises about the patient safety
- Review study related issues or problem and recommend appropriate solution for these issues

For more detail on the study committees, see Chapter 7.

Protocol Deviations This section includes discussion on how protocol deviations will be reported, to whom they will be reported, and how serious protocol deviations will be managed by the sponsor. Protocol deviations should be defined in the protocol and classified into:

- Inclusion/exclusion criteria deviation
- Protocol procedure deviations
- Compliance issues deviations
  - Missing follow-up visits
  - Issues associated with the ICF

Record Retention This section will discuss for how long the records of the study will be kept at the study sites. If international clinical sites are participating in the study, then record retention time should be mentioned according to their regulations (if the time period is not shorter than that required by US regulations).

Study Reports Types of study reports—interim study reports, annual progress report, and final clinical report—, and the responsibility of the sponsor and study investigators for the preparation and completion of these reports are discussed in this section.

References The list of all references cited in the protocol should include the names of all authors, titles of articles, names of journals, and dates of publication.

Attachments Attachments to the protocol should include a informed consent form (ICF) template, and research contract templates, besides the case report forms (CRFs).

CASE REPORT FORMS (CRFs)

Study case report forms (CRFs) are defined as a printed, optical, or electronic collection instrument designed for clinical trial data capture. CRFs are designed to capture the data as described in the clinical protocol. During the course of the study, CRFs are monitored to ensure accuracy of reported data in accordance with source documentation of the data. The purpose for designing CRFs in a clinical study can be summarized as follow:

1. To ensure data collection was done in accordance with the study protocol
2. To fulfill the regulatory authority requirements for data collection
3. To facilitate effective, comprehensive data processing and analysis of the results reported in a clinical study

CRFs are usually designed as printed hard copy or electronic CRFs. If printed hard copy are used, copies of all CRFs should be collected by the sponsor after the completion of the monitoring of the CRFs and then entered into the study database system. Electronic CRFs are starting now to be widely used, and this type of CRF requires extensive training on the electronic CRFs system prior to initiating the study. However, the study monitoring visits must be conducted whether printed hard copy or electronic CRFs are used. It is always good practice that the sponsor provide annotated CRFs when printed CRFs are used or description of each data field for electronic CRFs so that every item in the CRFs's defined. Providing instructions of the CRFs to the study sites may reduce the monitoring time and the number of queries regarding inconsistencies in the study.

To facilitate effective, comprehensive data processing and analysis, it is also recommended that when developing the protocol-derived questions, those questions that require answers in narrative or lengthy text format be avoided as much as possible, and instead the CRFs be designed to respond to questions in the check box format. An example is information gathered on investigational product failure or a malfunction event. Check boxes that relate to various device component failure events would facilitate data processing, and spaces requiring narratives about device malfunction or failure incidents would not.

In global clinical studies, where international sites are participating in the study, and the final clinical report is probably going to be submitted to the FDA as well as other regulatory bodies, early communication is encouraged with the US and the international teams to coordinate the CRFs and to provide alternative unit definitions, and thus to instruct investigators on which units to use to avoid confusion of units. For example, the units of certain items should be defined, such as weight (lb or kg), height (in or cm), blood glucose (mg/dl, or mM), and whether these parameters are specified by a single unit system.

General Instructions for Completing and Correcting Study Case Report Forms

- The investigator must ensure the accuracy, legibility, and completeness of data entry in the case report forms (CRFs) and in all other required report forms/logs.
- Only authorized study staff (name shown in authorized signatory form) are allowed to enter data into the CRF and other required report forms.
- Ballpoint pen must be used (for printed CRFs).
- All items must be completed by entering a number or text in the space provided.
- When a subject is recruited into the trial, the initial and allocated numbers are entered in the CRF against the subject's name on the Subject Identification Code List. The subject's name should never be entered in the CRF to preserve confidentiality.
- The CRF should be completed during subject participation.
- Data reported on the CRFs that are derived from source documents should be consistent with the source documents, or the discrepancies should be explained.

Case Report Form Corrections

- Only authorized study staff can make corrections.
- Do not allow the clinical monitor/sponsor to make correction in the CRF.
- Corrections should not obscure the original entry (for printed CRFs):
  - Do not erase.
  - Do not overwrite.
  - Never use correcting fluids.
- To make a correction (for printed CRFs):
  - Cross out the wrong entry with a single line.
  - Write the correct entry alongside/above/under the wrong entry.
  - Date the correction.
  - Initial the correction.
  - Explain the correction (if necessary).

Sections of the CRFs   It should be stressed that the structure and material subject of CRFs depend ultimately on the data to be collected in accordance with the study protocol. The following is a universal outlines of CRFs:

Screening and Enrollment CRF
- Subjects' inclusion and exclusion criteria
- Subjects' demographics (sex, age, race, highest, weight, etc.)
- Baseline assessments (physical, clinical history, medications, lab tests, imaging tests, etc.)

CRF Procedure
- Investigational device accountability
- Device malfunction/failure
- Measured procedure parameters

Follow-Up CRFs
- Specific tests or measurements
- Report of adverse events

Adverse Events CRFs
- Description of the AE, including signs and symptoms of adverse events
- Whether the adverse is serious adverse event (SAE). If the adverse event is designated as SAE, then specify the basis of this determination.
- Whether the adverse events relate to study procedure
- Whether the adverse events related to study device
- Whether the adverse event is unanticipated
- Start, stop date of the AE, or record if the adverse still ongoing
- Outcome of the adverse event (i.e., resolved, unresolved, ongoing, or resolved with residual effect)
- Severity or strength of the adverse event (i.e., mild, moderate, or severe)

Protocol Deviations CRFs
- Inclusion/exclusion criteria deviations
- Study procedure deviations
- Study compliance deviations (e.g., missing visit deviations and deviations associated with the ICF)

Study Completion Data in CRF
- Whether subject completed or did not complete study. If subject did not complete the study, then give the reasons for not completing the study: subjects expires (give expiration date if known), subject lost to follow-up (give date of subject lost to follow-up and closest follow-up visit), or subject withdrew consent (give date of subject's withdrawal from study)
- Signature of the PI
- Signature of the person who completed the CRFs

Source Documents

Documents that could be viewed as source documents in a clinical trial include the following:

- Subject medical file
- Medical and medication history
- Instrument printouts
- Laboratory results
- Product dispensing records, accountability
- Laboratory notes
- Physician notes
- Nurse notes

EXAMPLE OF THE CASE REPORT FORM TEMPLATE

The following case report form templates are examples of the type of information that should be included in the forms. However, the exact information used in CRFs is dependent on the study protocol.

SCREENING/ENROLLMENT CASE REPORT FORM

Protocol Title and Number:
Case Report Forms Number and Version:
Patient ID: _____
Patient Initials: ___ ____ ____
Date: ____/____/____
      MM DD YY

Section 1—Enrollment

Inclusion Criteria

All of the following criteria must be marked *YES* for the patient to be enrolled in the study:

NO	YES	N/A	Inclusion Criteria
☐	☐	☐	
☐	☐	☐	
☐	☐	☐	
☐	☐	☐	
☐	☐	☐	

Exclusion Criteria

All of the following criteria must be marked *NO* for the patient to be enrolled in the study:

NO	YES	N/A	
☐	☐	☐	
☐	☐	☐	
☐	☐	☐	
☐	☐	☐	

Section 2—Demographics

Date of Birth: ___/___/___
              mm dd yy

Gender: ☐ Male   ☐ Female

Height: _____   ☐ inches   ☐ cm   ☐ Not evaluated

Weight: _____   ☐ lb   ☐ kg   ☐ Not evaluated

Race:

☐ White

☐ Black

☐ American Indian

☐ Hispanic

☐ Asian

☐ Other

Section 3—Baseline Medical History
____ Check here if no medical history to report

Medical Condition	Start Date	End Date or Ongoing

Section 4—Physical Exam

Body System	Normal	Abnormal	Comment If Abnormal	Not Evaluated
Skin				
Lymphatic				
Eyes, Ears, Nose, Throat				
Neck				
Respiratory				
Cardiovascular				
Gastrointestinal				
Musculoskeletal				
Neurological				

Section 5—Medication(s) Used

Name of the Medication	Start Date	Stop Date	Ongoing	Dose and Route of Administration

Section 6—Principal Investigator's Verification of Subject Eligibility

YES	NO	
☐	☐	Did the subject meet all qualifications for participation in the study?

Section 7—Signatures

Date: ___/___/___
    mm dd yy
Signature of Investigator: _____
Signature of Person Completing Form: _____

INFORMED CONSENT FORM (ICF)[3]

The following important issues should be prepared when developing an informed consent template:

- Subject consenting is a process by which a subject voluntarily confirms his/her willingness to participate in a particular clinical study, after having been informed of all aspects of the clinical study that are relevant to the subject's decision to participate.
- Every subject participating in a clinical study must sign an ICF prior to participation in the study (in some cases the legal representative of the patient signs the ICF).
- The person who is discussing the ICF with the patient must also sign this form.
- To prove that ICF was signed prior to participation in the study, this form may include the date and time of signing the consent form.
- If the subject can't provide a signed ICF because of a certain medical condition, then the ICF should be signed by the legal representative of the subject.
- Certain clinical studies are waived from obtaining ICF based on the urgency of the study and the condition of the subject. The waiver from consenting the subject must be approved by the FDA.
- The ICF should be administered to subject in the subject's own language.
- The ICF should be administered to subject in layperson language where scientific terms are simplified as much as possible.

Elements of the ICF (21 CFR 50)

The elements of the ICF as identified in 21 CFR 50.25 can be summarized as follows:

- A statement that the study involves research
- An explanation of purpose of the research
- An explanation of number of sites, and number of patients to be enrolled in the study
- A description of expected duration of the study, and patients' follow-up visits
- A discussion of the experimental procedures to be followed

- A description of any reasonably foreseeable risks or discomforts to the subjects
- A description of the benefits to subjects, or to others, expected from the research
- A disclosure of specific, appropriate alternative procedures or courses of treatment, if any, that might be available to the subjects
- A statement informing the subjects that their medical records may be examined by the sponsor, FDA, or other regulatory bodies, and the extent to which those records will be kept confidential
- An explanation as to whether any compensation or medical treatment is available if injury occurs
- An explanation of whom to contact for answers to pertinent questions:
  - About the research
  - About research subject's rights
  - About any research-related injury
- A statement that participation is voluntary, with no penalty or loss of benefits to which the subject is otherwise entitled
- A statement that particular treatment or procedures may involve risks to the embryo or fetus, if the subject is or becomes pregnant, that are currently unforeseeable
- A statement of anticipated circumstances under which a subject's participation may be discontinued by the investigator without regard to the subject's consent
- A statement that significant new findings developed during the course of the research that may relate to the subject's willingness to continued participation will be provided to the subject
- Informed consent requirements do not preempt federal, state, or local laws
- A physician has the ultimate authority for the patient's emergency care to the extent that the physician is permitted under applicable federal state or local laws

Challenges of Writing an Informed Consent Document

Two main challenges encountered when writing the informed consent document: readability and subject's understanding of content of this consent.

Readability: The following readability issues should be taken into consideration when writing the consent:

- Document should be easily understandable
- Use 8th grade reading writing level
- Define all technical terms e.g. "Catheter" is a small plastic tube
- Provide explicit information
- Give concrete examples
- Demonstrate clear purpose
- Use mental images when a possible

Comprehension

- Shorten words by removing unnecessary prefixes and suffixes, using simple synonyms
- Average readable sentence length in American English is 17 words long
- Sentences are considered too long if they contain more than 30 words
- Organization and Visual Presentation:
  - Organize content under topical headings or short questions
  - Appropriate use of illustrations can improve comprehension

Monitoring of the Informed Consent

Issues/problems are frequently identified during monitoring visits regarding the informed consent include the following:

- Consent forms not dated by the subject
- Consent forms not signed and/or dated by the investigator or consent designee
- Consent forms not signed and/or dated by a witness (when applicable)
- Use of an expired consent form or different version from the IRB currently approved version
- Consent form signed by a consent designee not authorized by the IRB
- Dates for subject's signature and that of the investigator or consent designee do not match on the consent form

Exception from ICF Requirement

Exception from the ICF requirements may include the following situations:

- Life-threatening situation necessitating use of the test article
- ICF cannot be obtained because of inability to communicate with, or obtain legally effective consent from the subject
- Time is not sufficient to obtain consent from the subject's legal representative
- No alternative method of approval or generally recognized therapy is available that provides an equal or greater like hood of saving the subject's life.

Exception from ICF for Planned Emergency Research[4,5]

In planned emergency research where the subject is unable to provide consent, the ICF can be waived by the FDA.

INSTRUCTIONS FOR USE OF DEVICE

This document includes all device instructions for use for clinical users. It includes the following sections:

- Device description
- Indication(s)
- Contraindications
- Potential adverse events
- Warnings
- Risks
- Precautions
- Directions for use
- Storage and handling

Device Description   The detailed description of the device should include diagrams and photographs as needed.

Indication(s)   The intended use of the device should give the patient population and intended disease or condition to be treated.

Contraindications   A list of certain conditions where the device cannot be used or the use of the device will be harmful to the patient, should note how this item can be sometimes mistakenly used and cite the precautions. Contraindications mean that device cannot be technically used because of a patient anatomy or disease condition, whereas precautions mean that device can be either used with caution or not used because of complications that can occur in certain disease conditions.

Potential Adverse Events   List of all anticipated adverse events that can be related to the study product or study procedures.

Warnings   List any special device warnings that the clinical users should be aware of.

Risks   Discuss any potential risks associated with the use of the device (precautions: special precautions and monitoring procedures that the clinical users should be made aware of).

Directions for Use   Procedural use of the device should be given step by step.

Storage and Handing   List conditions for the device's storage, such as temperature, humidity, and light.

STUDY REGULATORY BINDER

This file contains all regulatory and administrative documents of the clinical study. The file also contains the various versions of the protocol, ICF, CRFs, and so forth. Copies of the study regulatory binder are kept at the study site and by the sponsor. The contents of the study regulatory binder consist of the following documents:

Study-Related Exhibits

- FDA study approval letters
- IRB Certificate of Approval issued by the IRB
- IRB approved informed consent documents
- HIPAA authorization form
- Investigator drug brochure/investigational device brochure

- FDA Form 1572 (Investigative New Drug Studies)
- Laboratory documents (lab certificates—e.g., CLIA, CAP, and normal value ranges)

Research Personnel Information
- Curriculum vitae: An updated CV of the investigator and co-investigator (within 12 months of submission)
- Medical license
- Financial disclosure
- Human research protection certification
- Study research contract (RC): A copy of the final signed research contract and amendment(s) of this contract

Study Tracking Logs
- Screening log
- Delegation of authority log
- Device accountability log
- Monitor visits log
- Training log
- Device shipment records

Study Correspondence
- Sponsor correspondence
- IRB correspondence

Study Clinical Materials
- Different approved versions of the study protocol
- Different approved versions of the CRFs
- Informed consent form (ICF) template and all approved IRB approved versions of the ICF
- Advertisements for the study that are approved by the IRB
- Instructions for use (IFU), or the investigator brochure
- Training materials including the initiation visit presentation

STUDY RESEARCH AGREEMENT

Contract's Structure

The research contract includes the following categories and provisions:

- General provisions
- Special provisions
- Miscellaneous provisions
- Exhibits and addenda

General Provisions
- Scope of work (study protocol)
- Personnel (principal investigator and sub-investigators)
- Duration (enrollment period)
- Data record keeping and access (case report forms)
- Communications (institution and sponsor contacts)
- IRB approval (informed consent form [ICF], and HIPAA regulation)
- Independent contractor who is not part of sponsor
- Use of name (authorized name of sponsor and clinical sites)

Special Provisions
- Cost and payment terms: incentives (enrollment and time targets), administrative fees (department and university overhead), and infrastructure costs (IRB, advertising, pharmacy)
- Confidential information
- HIPAA compliance
- Publication rights
- Intellectual property rights
- Indemnification of institution and principal investigator by sponsor
- Subject injuring compensation
- Insurance
- Financial disclosure of participating investigators

Miscellaneous Provisions
- Governing and controlling federal and state laws
- Amendments and severability
- Assignment
- Return of investigational product
- Terms of record retention
- Debarment warranty

Exhibits and Amendments
- Itemized cost breakdown
- Schedule of payments
- Clinical protocol

Confidentiality

This item obligates institution, principal investigators, and sub-investigators to maintain sponsor information in confidence for the specified period of time in the contract. However, this does not apply to information that is:

- In the public domain
- Known to institution or principal investigator before start of study
- Disclosed by a third party with a right to do so
- Required by law to be disclosed
- Necessary to assure proper medical care

Publication Rights

The investigator is free to publish methods/data/results of study after multi-center publication but subject to prior review by sponsor. The Sponsor, however, has:

- Time-limited right of review (usually 30 days or more)
- No right to withhold publication
- No editorial control
- Direct multi-center publication

Intellectual Property Rights

The sponsor's inventions are protected by patent, copyright, and trade secrets related to the sponsor's study drug/device/biologic and based on the sponsor's confidential information. The Institution' inventions are:

- Protected by patent or copyright
- Invented by the institution's employee

- Not directly related to study drug/device/biologic (or new formulation, indication, use)
- Not based on the sponsor's confidential information

Joint Inventions are:

- Invented by employees of the institution and the sponsor
- Joint ownership with right to license

Indemnification

The sponsor should indemnify for any injuries arising from the study. The indemnification provision relieves the institution (subsidiaries, affiliates, officers, trustees, etc.), principal investigators and sub-investigators of any liability resulting from the use or administration of the study drug/device/biologic or arising from a study-required procedure provided that:

- Protocol instructions of sponsor are followed without serious protocol violations
- Informed consent is obtained from the study patient
- All applicable FDA or other government requirements are followed
- No negligence or willful misconduct on part of principal investigator or Institution

RESEARCH AGREEMENT TEMPLATE

CLINICAL TRIAL SITE AGREEMENT

Clinical Study Title:
Protocol Number:
Effective Date:
Clinical Site Code:

RECITALS:

A. Sponsor of a clinical study is referred to as "Name of the Sponsor." This study is generally known as "INSERT TRIAL NAME HERE."

B. Institution, Primary Investigator, and Sponsor now desire to enter into an agreement to perform the Trial and, as part of that agreement, to set forth the respective rights and obligations of the parties, to establish the payment schedule for achievement of critical time points for this study.

NOW, THEREFORE, in consideration of the foregoing and the mutual promises herein contained, the parties agree as follows:

PARTIES TO AGREEMENT:

1. Sponsor: Name and Address of the Sponsor
2. Institution: Name and Address of the Site
3. Primary Investigator: Name and Address of the Site PI
4. Payment Information: Institution or Individual to whom
                         payment should be made (Trial Site):
                         Payee: _____
                         Mailing Address: _____
                         City/ State/ Zip: _____
                         Phone:_____
                         Federal Tax I.D. # (Social Security #
                         required if Payee is an Individual): _____

The parties hereby agree to the following terms of this Site Agreement:

(A) Total number of patients to be enrolled in the Trial:
(B) Estimated Start Date:
(C) Estimated enrollment Completion Date:
(D) Estimated completion of subject follow-up:
(E) Other provisions:

1. *Performance of the Trial*
Primary Investigator(s)/Institution agree to conduct the Trial in strict accordance with the Protocol, all applicable Food and Drug Administration ("FDA") regulations as written in the Code of Federal Regulations ("CFR"), including 21 CFR Part 56 and all applicable federal, state, and local laws, regulations, and guidelines relevant to the conduct of clinical medical device studies, all conditions imposed by the Institutional Review Board ("IRB").

Primary Investigator(s) shall obtain the approval of the IRB or similar committee formally designated by the Institution to review biomedical research, in conformance with the Guidelines. Primary Investigator(s) shall ensure that each patient enrolling in the Trial shall give his/her written informed consent, and that a copy of a written informed consent form be given to each participating patient or the participant's family, as appropriate in compliance with the Guidelines.

During the term of this Agreement, Sponsor may provide to Institution and Primary Investigator(s), or Institution and Primary Investigator(s) may generate, certain confidential and proprietary information, that belongs to Sponsor ("Confidential Information"). Primary Investigator(s) and Institution each acknowledge that all information, clinical or technical, including the operations manual, Protocol, forms and reports provided or generated during this Trial, is Confidential Information. Institution and Primary Investigator(s) each acknowledge and recognize the valuable and proprietary nature of the Confidential Information and agree that the Confidential Information shall remain the property of Sponsor. Except as otherwise provided in this Agreement, Institution and Primary Investigator(s) each agree to receive and maintain the Confidential Information in confidence and to refrain from any use thereof in whole or in part except for the express purpose authorized in this Agreement, without the express written permission of Sponsor. The limitations on disclosure and use of the Confidential Information shall survive for a period of five (5) years from the date of this Agreement.

Institution and Primary Investigator(s) each understand and agree that all data and results of this Trial are Confidential Information and may not be shared with or disseminated to any third party or combined with data or results of any other trial without the consent of Sponsor.

Primary Investigator(s) and Institution shall inform Sponsor of any serious adverse event, unanticipated adverse effect, any device failure, withdrawal of IRB approval, deviations from the investigational plan set forth in the Protocol, or any audit or inquiry into the Trial by any governmental authority, immediately but no later than twenty-four (24) hours after learning of such an event or occurrence. A full written report, by the Primary Investigator, of all the above-mentioned categories should be submitted to the Sponsor no later than ten (10) working days after learning of such event or occurrence.

2. *Individually Identifiable Health Information*
Institution and Primary Investigator(s) acknowledge and agree that the Health Insurance Portability and Accountability Act of 1996, P.L. 104-191, Subtitle F, and regulations from time to time promulgated thereunder ("HIPAA" or the "Privacy Rule"), require that Institution and/ or Primary Investigator(s), as a "covered Entity" under the Privacy Rule, obtain a signed authorization from a patient prior to using or

disclosing such patient's "Protected Health Information," as defined in the Privacy Rule, obtained or created in connection with the Trial. All parties agree to use and disclose Protected Health Information only in a manner consistent with the requirement of the Privacy Rule and any applicable patient authorization, including the terms and conditions of the Informed Consent and Authorization executed by each patient, or as otherwise may be permitted or required by applicable law.

3. *Record Keeping/Retention*
Primary Investigator(s)/Institution agree to maintain complete and up-to-date Trial records during the Trial including Case Report Forms and the Trial Site files, which includes all Trial-related correspondence. Primary Investigator(s)/ Institution agree to sign a statement in each patient's Case Report Form attesting that the data contained therein are an accurate accounting of the treatment, care, and events surrounding the patient's involvement in the Trial.
Primary Investigator(s)/Institution will retain all records for this Trial for the last to expire of:

(a) Two (2) years after the FDA approves the premarket Approval Application ("PMA")
(b) Two (2) years following the termination or withdrawal of the health regulatory agency exemption (e.g., Investigational Device Exemption ["IDE"] application) under which the Trial was conducted
(c) As defined by local, state and federal law and regulations; or

To avoid any possible errors, Primary Investigator(s)/Institution will contact Sponsor prior to the destruction of records or in the event of accidental loss or destruction of any Trial records.

4. *Sponsor's Right of Inspection*
Personnel from Sponsor (or its representatives) may call on Primary Investigator(s)/ Institution periodically at mutually convenient times to monitor and/or audit the Trial and answer procedural questions. Primary Investigator(s) and/or Institution agree, as defined in the Protocol, to make all Trial records and Trial participants' medical records available for comparison and/or copying if requested by Sponsor (or its representatives). Primary Investigator(s) and/or Institution also agree to cooperate with representatives of the FDA or any other regulatory agency in the event of an inspection of this Trial, and will provide the regulatory agency representative access to the above-described records.

5. *Liability/Insurance/Warranty Disclaimer*

The Primary Investigator(s) and Institution (which shall include their employees, agents, and representatives) each agree to be solely responsible for their negligent or reckless acts or omissions in the performance of their duties hereunder, and shall be financially and legally responsible for all liabilities, costs, damages, expenses, and attorney fees resulting from, or attributable to any and all such acts and omissions. Sponsor shall indemnify the Primary Investigator(s) and Institution (including their employees, agents and representatives, the "Indemnified Parties") from and against any product liability claims relating to the investigational device in the Trial, provided that this indemnity will not extend to any liability, damage, cost, or expense arising from the failure of the Indemnified Parties to adhere to the Protocol or the negligence or willful misconduct of the Indemnified Parties.

The Primary Investigator(s) and Institution each represent and warrant that they have a sufficient general and malpractice insurance program (on either an indemnity or self-insured basis to fully perform their responsibilities hereunder.

Sponsor will be responsible for reasonable unanticipated emergent patient medical care costs that are a direct result of a patient's participation in this Trial that are not covered by third party payors and that are not the result of negligence, failure to follow the Protocol or any reckless or willful malfeasance by Institution, Primary Investigators, or their employees, agents, officers, assigns, or other affiliated persons.

The Primary Investigator(s) and Institution each understand and agree that the Trial device is experimental in nature and that no warranty, either expressed or implied, is made by Sponsor or any other party regarding the device.

6. *Use of Name/Publicity/Scientific Publications*

No party shall, without the prior written consent of the affected party, use in advertising, publicity, or otherwise, the name, trademark, logo, symbol, or other image of the affected party including without limitation, any of such relating to Sponsor or any of its subsidiaries. The Primary Investigator(s) and Institution (which shall include their employees, agents, and representatives) will not issue or disseminate any press release or statement, nor initiate any communication of information regarding this Trial whether in written or oral form, to the media or third party without the prior written consent of Sponsor.

Sponsor acknowledges that it intends to publish a multi-center publication regarding the Trial results. The publication of the principal results from any single site experience within the Trial is not allowed until both the preparation and publication of the multi-center results. The Primary Investigator(s) and/or Institution may publish information or data collected or produced as a result of its participation in this Trial in appropriate scientific journals or other professional publications provided that drafts of the material are delivered to Sponsor for purposes of review and comment at least sixty (60) days prior to the first submission for publication or public release. No publication or presentation of the data or results of the Sponsor Trial may be presented until Sponsor determines that the database for the Trial is clean and locked and, that the primary and secondary endpoint analyses are consistent with the Protocol.

In all publications, credits shall be given to Sponsor for its sponsorship of the Trial and the supply of the device under the Trial. Upon successful completion of this Trial and eventual commercialization of the device, Sponsor will provide Primary Investigator(s)/Institution appropriate recognition of their contribution.

7. Termination of Agreement or Termination of a Party's Participation in Agreement

Any party has the right at any time, within thirty (30) days prior written notice to each of the other parties, to terminate this Agreement for any cause or no cause. In the event of premature termination of this Trial, the Primary Investigator(s)/Institution will be reimbursed appropriately for patients enrolled up to the date of termination for whom the CDMS receives a properly completed Case Report Form. No payment will be made to Primary Investigator(s)/Institution if the Trial is terminated at this Trial Site because Primary Investigator(s)/Institution did not adhere to the Protocol or this Agreement or if the Primary Investigator(s)/Institution terminate this Agreement without cause.

Primary Investigator(s)/Institution will contact Sponsor should one or more Primary Investigator(s) leave the Institution where the Trial is being conducted so that the records for this Trial can either be transferred to another party within the Institution or taken with the departing Primary Investigator(s), at the sole discretion of Sponsor.

8. Intellectual Property

All intellectual property rights in any discoveries, inventions, and/or enhancements reduced to practice by Primary Investigator(s) or Institution as a result of their performance of this Trial shall be assigned to Sponsor or its designee by Primary Investigator(s) and/or Institution. Primary Investigator(s)/Institution will cooperate with

Sponsor in Sponsor's 's patent and other filings and documentation relating thereto.

9. *Miscellaneous*

Primary Investigator(s)/Institution are operating as independent contractor(s) under this Agreement and not as agent(s) or employee(s) of Sponsor.

Primary Investigator(s) and/or Institution, by signing below, each warrant and represent that neither they nor any member of their immediate family (defined as spouse and children) have any real or perceived conflict of interest in the execution of this Trial (e.g., stock or other equity in companies that manufacture the device being tested in this Trial) and that participation herein does not conflict with any other obligation to third parties.

This Agreement and the Investigator Agreement set forth the entire agreement and understanding between the parties relating to the Trial and supersedes and merges all prior discussions, correspondence, negotiations, and agreements between them relating thereto. In the event of any conflict between the terms of this Agreement and the Investigator Agreement, the terms of this Agreement shall control.

Except as otherwise provided herein, this Agreement may not be amended, supplemented, or otherwise modified except by an instrument in writing signed by all parties to be bound.

The parties have consented to the terms of this Agreement by signing below. Each party should retain one copy of this Agreement for their records. The *original* must be returned to Sponsor:

PRIMARY INVESTIGATOR:

_____

Name and Title (print or type)

_____   _____

Signature   Date

INSTITUTION:

_____

Name and Title (print or type)

_____   _____

Signature   Date

Sponsor Corporation:

_____

Name and Title (print or type)

_____   _____

Signature   Date

RESEARCH CONTRACT CHALLENGES

Contract signing is one of the latest steps in approving clinical studies and this document is usually executed just prior to initiating the study. Sufficient time should be planned in advance to complete this activity, especially if the selected site is an academic institution because several personnel have to review and sign the contract. The budget for the research should be appropriately set up to cover the expenses of the research, institution overhead cost, subject re-imbursement, administrative cost, and research staff cost. The research expenses should be limited to research procedures that are not covered by the standard of care. For multicenter trials, negotiation with the cost of research procedures starts with the Medicare prices for these procedures. Subject re-imbursement includes the cost of travel of the subject and any re-imbursement associated with time spent on research activities to provide responses to specific study questionnaires. Institution overhead cost is usually constant and institution dependent. Administrative costs include expenses for advertisement for the study, mail, coping, and other appropriate costs. The IRB cost for the study is usually set up as direct billing from the IRB to the sponsor.

Challenges to the research contract of a clinical study could exist in four categories of the contract:

- Indemnification
- Publication policy
- Insurance
- Subject's injury

Indemnification: The contract should specify whether the sponsor will or will not indemnify, or whether the sponsor is requesting mutual indemnification. It is usually stated in the contract that the site will not incur liability by the normal course of business, any provision of service in connection with study, and sponsor's indemnification in case of manufacturing defect of the study product.

Insurance: The sponsor should carry minimum levels of insurance and prove liquid assets to cover liabilities which are mainly determined by the risk of the study.

Publication: The research contract usually allows for 30–60 day publication review and may include other terms for publication restriction, or approval.

Subject's Injury: The contract includes a paragraph about subject injury reimbursement that is not related to physician negligence.

CLINICAL FORMS AND CERTIFICATES

Several clinical forms and certificates are needed for a clinical study, including financial disclosure form or certificate, screening log, site communication log, site training log, monitoring visit log, site delegation of authority log, and device inventory log. The financial disclosure form is required for the sponsor to evaluate whether investigators have a conflict of interest in conducting the research; the other forms are required to document management, training, and monitoring of the study.

Financial Disclosure Certificate[6,7]

The financial disclosure certificate or form is completed for every investigator and sub-investigator involved in the study. The form is evaluated by the sponsor for any conflict of interest issues among the investigators:

- The investigators covered are any principal investigator or sub-investigator directly involved in the treatment and evaluation of the research subjects
- Completion of this form is also required for studies that support the submission of Investigational Device Exemption (IDE), Pre-Market Approval (PMA), Humanitarian Device Exemption (HDE), or Pre-Market Notification [510 (K)].

The elements of the financial disclosure are as follows:

- Disclose any financial arrangement entered into between the sponsor of the covered study and clinical investigators involved in the conduct of the study, whereby the value of compensation to investigator for conducting the study could be influenced by the outcome of the study.

- Disclose any significant payments of other sorts from the sponsor of covered study, such as a grant to fund ongoing research, compensation in form of equipment, retainer for ongoing consultation, or honoraria (whose value exceeds $25,000.00).
- Disclose any proprietary interest in the tested product held by any clinical investigator involved in a study.
- Disclose any significant equity interest in the sponsor of covered study held by any clinical investigator involved in any clinical study (whose value exceeds $50,000 in a publicly traded company).
- Recognize any steps taken to minimize the potential for bias resulting from any of the disclosed arrangements, interests, or payments.

Clinical Forms

1. Screening Log
2. Site Communication Log
3. Site Training Log
4. Monitoring Visit Log
5. Site Delegation of Authority Log
6. Device Inventory Log

Site Communications Log   This log contains the communications between the sponsor and investigational site: any communications regarding adverse events, procedure instructions, monitor visits, and so forth, should be kept in this log. This log contains the following items:

- Site ID number
- Type of communication (e-mail, telephone call, etc.)
- Date of communication
- Name of the person received or sent the communication
- Description of the communication

Patient Screening Log   This log includes a list of all screened subjects, including screen failure subjects and reasons why subjects were not enrolled in the study. This log is created to ensure that an unbiased adequate number of suitable subjects is selected as defined in the protocol. This document also defines the criteria for screen failure subjects for not being enrolled in the study. This information can be utilized, upon modifying certain criteria, to increase subject enrollment if the enrollment is slow in the trial. This log contains the following items:

- Site ID number
- Patient ID number
- Did patient meet inclusion/exclusion, and baseline assessment criteria? (yes or no)
- Did patient enrolled in the study? (yes or no)
- Date of enrollment

Monitor Visit Log   This log is used to document study monitoring visits and contains the following items:

- Site ID number
- Visitor name
- Title
- Type of visit
- Date of the visit
- Signature of the monitor

Site Delegation of Authority Log   The delegation of authority of sub-investigators or other research staff by the PI is filled in this log as follows:

- Site ID number
- Name of the delegate
- Date of the delegation
- Responsibility of the delegate
- Delegate signature
- PI signature

Site Training Log   Site training is documented in this log as follows:

- Site ID number
- Name and title of the trainee
- Name and title of the person(s) providing training

- Date of the training visit
- Signature of the trainee

Device Inventory Log The investigator should account for device received, used, or returned from the sponsor in accordance with the clinical protocol. This is an administrative log to keep an overview of investigational device received, used, or returned by the investigational site:

- Device shipped
- Device used
- Device returned

CLINICAL STANDARD OPERATING PROCEDURES (SOPs)

Clinical standard operating procedures (SOPs) refer to the specific procedures developed by the sponsor for the Investigator to follow in conducting, managing, and executing clinical projects and studies. At a minimum, the clinical SOPs should cover certain clinical processes, such as, reporting of adverse events, Interim monitoring procedures, development of the ICF template, development of the clinical protocol, and master clinical file contents. Clinical SOPs can be developed by the study sponsor, or CRO (contract research organization) if a CRO is contracted for the study. It is important to document which SOP is being followed at every phase of the clinical study. For example, for qualification of study investigators/study sites, and for interim monitoring visits, the sponsor should determine whether the investigators followed their own procedures or the contracted CRO's SOP.

SOP Contents

The clinical SOP generally contains the following sections:

- *Purpose* The clear aim of each procedure should be stated, such as the procedures developed for reporting of adverse events during the course of a clinical study.
- *Scope of the procedure* This section should describe the type of study in which the developed procedures will be applied and the limitations of the procedure.

- *Definitions*   Certain technical items and processes listed in the SOP are clarified in this section, such as case report forms and the clinical research associate's function.
- *Responsibilities*   The responsibilities of the departments, different teams, or individuals associated with the execution of each activity listed in the procedure are discussed in this section, such as those of the clinical manager, CRA, and regulatory manager.
- *Procedures Followed*   The procedures to be followed by the staff are discussed in this section, according to who performs what task, and with detailed description of the task.
- *Related References*   References to other SOPs, regulations, or publications are listed in this section.
- *Attachments*   Any special attachments that may be necessary are listed in this procedure.

Rationale for Developing Clinical SOPs

The rational for developing SOPs for certain clinical operations could be summarized as follows:

- Ensure that the sponsor has consistent processes that meet or even exceed regulatory and good clinical practice (GCP)
- Demonstrate that clinical research staff are familiar with these processes
- Ensure that processes are reviewed and updated on a regular basis
- Ensure that audits by the FDA do not result in serious findings

Sample SOPs

Three examples of sample SOPs are provided in this section to get familiar with the process of developing SOPs.

1. Standard Operating Procedure for Qualifying and Selection of Investigators and Clinical Sites	
Title:	Standard Operating Procedure for Qualifying and Selection of Investigators and Clinical Sites
Purpose:	The purpose of this SOP is to list the procedures and responsibilities for qualifying and selecting investigators/clinical sites for a clinical study.
Scope:	This SOP is applied to all clinical studies conducted by the sponsor: IDE feasibility, IDE pivotal and post-market studies.

1. Standard Operating Procedure for Qualifying and Selection of Investigators and Clinical Sites

Definitions: The following terms used in this SOP are defined as follow:

Clinical Affairs (CA)
A department of persons trained and experienced in the conduct of clinical studies. This group manages and oversees implementation and the overall progress of the clinical study, whether directly or by utilization of consultant(s) and/or CRO(s).

Clinical Site or Center
Any public or private entity or agency or medical or dental facility where clinical trials are conducted.

Contract Research Organization (CRO)
A person or an organization (academic, commercial, etc.) contracted by the sponsor to perform one or more of trial-related duties and/or functions.

Monitor
A person who has been trained to the investigational protocol(s), informed consent, instructions for use, applicable SOPs and regulatory requirements, who checks and reports the progress of the clinical study at an investigational site or other data gathering organization (e.g., core lab or other study facility). The monitor is designated by the sponsor and may be an employee, a consultant, or an employee of a consultant to a Contract Research Organization (CRO) retained by the sponsor. Throughout this document the person conducting the assessment/qualification site visit will be referred to as the "monitor."

Principal Investigator (PI)
An individual who actually conducts a clinical investigation, and under whose immediate direction the test article is administered or dispensed to, or used involving, a patient, or, in the event of an investigation conducted by a team of individuals, is the responsible leader of that team.

Clinical Research Coordinator (CRC)
Also may be referred to as Research Coordinator, Study Coordinator, Research Nurse, and so forth. This individual, who is under the direction of the PI, manages most of the administrative responsibilities for a clinical trial on behalf of the PI, frequently acts as a liaison between investigative site and sponsor, and reviews data and records prior to a monitor's site visit(s). The CRC may also perform and/or manage other study-specific duties as appropriately delegated by the PI.

Sub-Investigator (Sub-I)
An individual who is under the direction of the PI and performs specific clinical study-related activities.

1. Standard Operating Procedure for Qualifying and Selection of Investigators and Clinical Sites

Subject

May also be referred to as "patient" or "trial subject or patient." This individual participates in a clinical trial, either as a recipient of an investigational product or as a control.

Responsibilities:

1. The clinical study manager is responsible for preparing and providing a list of all potential investigators and sites for the study to the assigned clinical research associate.

2. The clinical research monitor who is assigned to the study is responsible for conducting the qualifying visit and completing the visit report.

3. The director of the clinical affairs department is responsible for finalizing the selection of the investigators and clinical sites from the list of qualified potential investigators who were evaluated for the study.

Procedures:

1. The clinical study manager is responsible for preparing and providing a list of all potential investigators and sites to the study monitors who will conduct the evaluation. The information in the list is compiled from multiple sources, including the marketing department, clinical advisors, other investigators, and publications, and include the names of investigators who have experience in certain research fields.

2. The monitor sends out a Confidentiality Agreement to be signed by the potential PI prior to exchanging information about the product and the study.

3. The monitor sends out the protocol synopsis to interested potential investigators.

4. The clinical research monitor schedules a qualifying study visit with the potential investigator.

5. The monitor completes the qualifying monitoring visit report, which includes an evaluation of the investigator, the research staff, and the facility.

6. The director of the clinical affairs department finalizes the investigator and site list from potentially qualified investigators.

7. The clinical study manager or designee sends out a letter to inform potential investigators whether or not they were selected for the study.

References:

21 CFR Part 812 FDA Investigational Device Exemption
ICH E6 Guideline for Good Clinical Practice

Attachments:

Qualifying Visit Questionnaire Template
Qualifying Visit Report Template

2. SOP for Reporting Adverse Events in a Clinical Study

Title: SOP for Reporting Adverse Events in a Clinical Study

Purpose: The purpose of this document is to define the methods and activities for adverse event reporting in the clinical studies conducted by the sponsor.

Scope: This procedure applies to all adverse events that occur during a clinical study conducted by the sponsor.

Definitions:

Clinical Affairs (CA)
A department of persons trained and experienced in the conduct of clinical studies. This group manages and oversees implementation and the overall progress of the sponsor clinical study, whether directly or by utilization of consultant(s) and/or CRO(s).

Clinical Site or Center
Any public or private entity or agency or medical or dental facility where clinical trials are conducted.

Monitor
A person who has been trained to the investigational protocol(s), informed consent, instructions for use, applicable SOPs and regulatory requirements, and who checks and reports the progress of the clinical study at an investigational site or other data gathering organization (e.g., core lab or other study facility). The monitor is designated by the sponsor and may be an employee, a consultant, or an employee of or consultant to a Contract Research Organization (CRO) retained by the sponsor. Throughout this document the person conducting the assessment/qualification site visit will be referred to as the "monitor."

Principal Investigator (PI)
An individual who actually conducts a clinical investigation, and under whose immediate direction the test article is administered or dispensed to, or used involving, a patient, or, in the event of an investigation conducted by a team of individuals, is the responsible leader of that team.

Subject
May also be referred to as "patient" or "trial subject or patient." An individual who participates in a clinical trial, either as a recipient of an investigational product or as a control.

2. SOP for Reporting Adverse Events in a Clinical Study

Case Report Forms (CRFs)
A printed, optical, or electronic collection instrument designed for clinical trial data capture.

Adverse Event (AE)
Any undesirable medical event occurring in a research subject, whether or not the event is considered related to the investigational device.

Serious Adverse Event (SAE)
An AE that results in death, a life-threatening condition (even if temporary in nature), hospitalization or prolonged hospitalization, a permanent impairment of body function or permanent damage to body structure, congenital anomaly/birth defect, or necessitates medical or surgical intervention to preclude permanent impairment of a body function or permanent damage to a body structure, or represents a serious medical event.

Anticipated Adverse Event
An AE that is listed in the clinical protocol or other study-related document that has been identified as a *potential* AE related to the investigational device or procedure being studied.

Unanticipated Adverse Device Effect (UADE)
Any serious adverse effect on health or safety or any life-threatening problem or death caused by, or associated with, a device, if that effect, problem or death was not previously identified in nature, severity, or degree of incidence in the investigational plan or application or any other unanticipated serious problem associated with a device that relates to the rights, safety, or welfare of subjects.

Responsibilities:

1. Clinical Affairs Management is responsible for interpretation, review, update, and implementation of this procedure.
2. Clinical Affairs Management is also responsible for the review of all adverse events case report forms and adverse event reports to ensure that these events were reported appropriately and within the time periods designated for reporting certain adverse events.
3. The Principal Investigator at the study site should report serious adverse events (SAEs) or unanticipated adverse device effects (UADE) to the sponsor within the designated time period described in the procedures section under this SOP.

2. SOP for Reporting Adverse Events in a Clinical Study

Procedures:

1. *Adverse Event Case Report Forms*   All adverse events must be recorded in the study adverse event case report forms. These forms include the following information about an adverse event:

   - Description of the AE, including signs and symptoms of the AE.
   - Whether or not the AE is a serious adverse event (SAE). If an adverse event is determined to be a SAE, then the rationale for this determination should be checked.
   - Whether the AE is anticipated or not. Anticipated AEs are listed in the study protocol as AEs which potentially could occur in the study.
   - Unanticipated adverse device effects. These are unexpected AEs which directly related to the study device.
   - Time onset and outcome of AE. This includes recording of the start date, stop date, or ongoing if the AE is not resolved. In addition, the outcome of the AE as to whether the event is resolved, not resolved, or resolved with sequelae, should be recorded in the AE-CRFs.
   - Relation of the AE to the study device. The relation of the AE to study device as to whether the event is related, possibly related, unrelated, or unknown, should be recorded in the AE-CRFs.
   - Relation of the AE to the study procedure. The relation of the AE to study procedures as to whether the event is related, possibly related, unrelated, or unknown, should be recorded in the AE-CRFs.
   - Adverse event severity. Adverse event severity/intensity should be classified as to whether the AE is mild, moderate, or severe.

2. *Adverse Events Reporting Time Periods*
   - Serious adverse events (SAEs) and serious UADE should be reported to the sponsor within 24 hours after the investigators are becoming aware of the event (this time period is determined by the sponsor). A final report of the SAEs and any serious UADE must be submitted to the sponsor no later than 10 working days after Investigators become aware of the event.
   - SAEs and the serious UADE should be reported to IRB in accordance with the institution's IRB policy.
   - If the UADE is judged to present *unreasonable risk* to subjects, the sponsor should suspend all studies presenting that risk, as soon as possible, but at most within 5 days after becoming aware of this risk. The sponsor must report these findings to FDA, IRBs, and participating Investigators within 10 working days.

2. SOP for Reporting Adverse Events in a Clinical Study

References:

    1. 21 CFR Part 812 FDA Investigational Device Exemption

    2. ICH E6 Guideline for Good Clinical Practice

    3. ISO 14155 Clinical Investigations of Medical Devices for Human Patients

Attachments:

    Adverse Event CRF Template

3. Standard Operating Procedure for the Development of Statistical Analysis Plan (SAP)

Title: Standard Operating Procedure for Development of Statistical Analysis Plan

Purpose: This standard operating procedure (SOP) describes the process for the development and maintenance of Statistical Analysis Plan for clinical studies.

Scope: This SOP is applied to all clinical studies conducted by the sponsor: IDE feasibility, IDE pivotal and post-market studies. This SOP will be used as guidance for the sharing of data across participant sites, and the regulatory community.

Definitions: The following terms used in this SOP are defined as follow:

Case Report Forms (CRFs)
A printed, optical, or electronic collection instrument designed for clinical trial data capture.

Clinical Protocol
A study plan on which all clinical trials are based. The plan is carefully designed to safeguard the health of the participants as well as answer specific research questions. A protocol describes what types of people may participate in the trial; the schedule of tests, procedures, medications, and dosages; and the length of the study. While in a clinical trial, participants following a protocol are seen regularly by the research staff to monitor their health and to determine the safety and effectiveness of their treatment

Clinical Protocol Amendment
Changes to the clinical protocol during the course of the study

Statistical Analysis Plan (SAP)
The Statistical Analysis Plan (SAP) refers to the procedures followed by the sponsor of the study to define and analyze the study endpoints, measurements, and also to discuss the basis for the sample size determination of the study. The detailed SAP includes a plan for how the data of the study is to be presented in tables, figures, and listings.

Data Manager
This person is responsible for the entry of the data of a clinical study into specific database system. This responsibility includes the final generation of the data of clinical study in the form of tables, graphs, and charts.

3. Standard Operating Procedure for the Development of Statistical Analysis Plan (SAP)

Responsibilities:

Study Statistician is responsible for:

1. Ensuring that the protocol and any amendments cover all relevant statistical issues clearly and accurately.
2. Reviewing the CRFs to ensure that primary and secondary endpoints are collected and/or captured appropriately to satisfy analyses called for in the SAP, where applicable.
3. Working with the clinical data manager to update the study plan if the SAP changes and if those changes reflect changes to data collected during the conduct of the clinical research trial.

Clinical Study Team
The entire clinical team involved in the study is responsible for providing input to the Study Statistician on the protocol and SAP.

Procedures:

1. The SAP is a clearly defined section within the protocol and approved prior to the start of clinical research study.
2. The SAP should include the details of the planned statistical analyses associated with a clinical study. The analyses are planned to include the desired work product(s) and to be conducted in a consistent and repeatable manner.
3. The SAP should contain the detailed requirements and parameters for the reporting results of the clinical research trial, the format and content of output reports, and the tests to support the robustness and sensitivity of the analysis conducted.
4. Recommended checks and specific monitoring procedures should implemented to ensure and improve the quality of the plan and the associated data, as well as prevent any study compromise.
5. The SAP should include, at a minimum, for each primary and secondary endpoint:
   - How the outcome will be measured.
   - Any transformations on the data likely to be required before analysis.
   - Appropriate statistical tests to be used to analyze the data.
   - How missing data will be accounted for in the analyses (both scientifically and statistically).
   - Whether statistical inference will be drawn and whether any statistical adjustments for multiple comparisons will be performed.

References: 21 CFR Part 11

Attachments: Attach any specific SAP documents

3

QUALIFICATION/SELECTION OF STUDY INVESTIGATORS AND STUDY MONITORING VISITS

This chapter deals with important tasks for clinical studies qualification and selection of investigators, clinical sites, site training, and study monitoring visits. The study monitoring visits are grouped according to the phase of the study. For example, the study initiation visit is conducted right before enrollment in the study is started, interim

Design, Execution, and Management of Medical Device Clinical Trials,
by Salah Abdel-aleem
Copyright © 2009 John Wiley & Sons, Inc.

monitoring visits are conducted periodically during the course of the study, and the study close-out visit is conducted after the completion of all follow-up visits in the study. In this chapter the study monitoring reports are discussed in a comparable manner to the type of conducted visit. This chapter includes a detailed discussion of the qualification and selection of study investigators and study sites. This chapter also explains the responsibilities of the study monitors in accordance with the type of site visit. The chapter ends with a presentation and examples of study monitoring reports.

QUALIFICATION AND SELECTION OF INVESTIGATORS

The qualification and selection of clinical investigators and study sites is one of the early activities for preparation of a clinical study. The objective of this process is to select investigators who have the experience, interest in participating in the study, and are able to execute the trial as planned. The potential investigator should be able to recruit patients within the projected time period for subject enrollment, and should have a qualified research team and adequate clinical research facility to carry out the research. The research team consists of sub-investigators and a clinical research staff member (e.g., a clinical research coordinator). The research facility should have the required diagnostic labs, imaging labs, space for storage of investigational product/study documents, and adequate monitoring space.

A list of potential investigators can be compiled from multiple sources, key among these being the marketing and sales groups of the sponsor, clinical advisors, other clinical investigators, and publications in the research field.

During the qualifying visit the sponsor representative evaluates the investigator, research staff, and the research facility for participation in the study. The sponsor should develop a questionnaire to evaluate the principal investigator and his/her clinical site. The outcome or feedback obtained from this questionnaire and visit (e.g., the completed Qualification Visit Questionnaire) and the evaluation of the principal investigator and sub-investigators should be kept in the study files to document this selection process.

Responsibilities of the Principal Investigator[8]

The responsibilities of the Principal Investigator in a medical device study are similar to the responsibilities of the PI listed on Form 1572 for drugs:

- Conduct the study in accordance with the relevant, current protocol.
- Make changes to a protocol (protocol deviations) only after notifying the sponsor, except when necessary to protect the safety, rights, or welfare of subjects.
- Personally conduct or supervise the described investigation.
- Inform patients, or any persons used as controls, that the device is being used for investigational purposes and ensure that the requirements relating to obtaining informed consent in 21 CFR Part 50 and institutional review board (IRB) review and approval in 21CFR Part 56 are met.
- Report to the sponsor adverse events that occur in the course of the investigation.
- Read and understand the information in the investigator's brochure, including the potential risks and potential adverse effects of the device.
- Ensure that all associates, colleagues, and employees assisting in the conduct of the study are informed about their obligations in meeting the above-noted commitments.
- Maintain adequate and accurate records and to make those records available for inspection.
- Ensure that an IRB that complies with the requirements of 21 CFR Part 56 will be responsible for the initial and continued review and approval of the clinical investigation. Agree to promptly report to the IRB all changes in the research activity and all unanticipated problems involving risks to human subjects or others. Additionally agree not to make any changes in the research without IRB approval, except where necessary to eliminate apparent immediate hazards to the human subjects.

The Qualification Visit Questionnaire

This questionnaire includes the following evaluations:

Investigator and Staff Review
- Is the investigator interested in conducting the study?
- Does the investigator have previous experience doing clinical research trials?
- Does the investigator have an adequate staff to conduct the study (including a dedicated clinical research coordinator)?

- Has the investigator ever been issued an FDA warning letter? What was the outcome of this warning?
- Is the investigator willing to conduct the study according to the described protocol?
- Are approvals other than local IRB/EC required at this site?
- Does the investigator have adequate access to the protocol's specified subject population?
- Will the investigator be conducting any other studies that will compete for a similar subject population?
- Does the investigator's name appear on the FDA (or other applicable regulatory body) debarment list?

Evaluation of Facilities
- Facilities, including laboratories and equipment, are adequate for safe and proper conduct of the study?
- Is there a suitable, dedicated and secure area for storage of investigational product?
- Is there a suitable, secure and dedicated area for storage of study documents, CRFs, etc.?
- Is there an adequate monitoring area?

Special Requirements for Certain Clinical Studies

Enrollment in some studies can proceed slowly if the right investigators cannot be found to manage patient enrollment. For example, the team of investigators of a study involving invasive clinical trials may need to include physicians from different specialization to manage study patients with left ventricular assist devices, percutaneous left ventricular assist devices, or percutaneous valve replacement devices. Although the clinical operator of such studies can be an interventional cardiologist or cardiac surgeon, physicians from various specializations would need to participate to manage the research (e.g., interventional cardiologist, cardiac surgeon, and heart failure physician), and thus to ensure optimal patient recruitment (and recruitment speed).

Another cause of slow enrollment in clinical trials may be the lack of patients with the condition to be studied. The author has experienced this problem with clinical trials designed to evaluate a left ventricular assist device for the treatment of cardiogenic shock. In such a case the sponsor could consider taking the following actions:

- Select a study center that has the specific patient population.
- Confirm that there is no other study competing for the available patient population.
- Conduct a pre-study survey with key investigators (10–20 investigators) to confirm the expected clinical effect of the investigational product (e.g., reduction of mortality by 10–20%) and other important assumptions of the study.
- Develop creative protocol that will limit the sample size of the study and prevent a lengthy enrollment period (e.g., the use of surrogate endpoints).
- Engage with the FDA at early stages of the trial to make the FDA aware of all the issues.

Communication with Potential Investigators

After completion of the qualification visit evaluation, a letter is sent out to evaluated potential investigators informing them whether or not they were selected for the study.

MONITORING VISITS

For any given clinical study, the number of monitors and the number of required monitoring visits is dependent on the following factors:

- Number and location of the clinical sites where the study is being conducted.
- Level of training and experience of the research staff at the clinical sites.
- Complexity of the study.
- Nature of the disease or other condition under study.

The number of monitoring visits is discussed later in this chapter in the section entitled "Study Monitoring Plan," where a plan is outlined to devote the adequate resources to monitor the study successfully.

Scheduling the Monitoring Visit

- Prior to the site visit, the monitor should provide written confirmation, such as the visit confirmation letter or a similarly worded document to the PI.

- This letter will conform to any requirements outlined in a study-specific Monitoring Plan.
- The letter will outline why, if anyone, will accompany the monitor: what staff is required to be present for the meeting, and what documents must be available for review by the monitor.
- Any outstanding issues from any previous visit(s) should be addressed during the upcoming visit.
- Ample time should be scheduled with the appropriate staff to discuss any issues or updates.
- Prior to the visit, any necessary documents and/or materials should be sent to the site.

Responsibilities of the Study Monitor

Qualified and experienced monitors should be assigned to monitor the study. To meet their several responsibilities during the preparation, execution, and management of the study through monitoring visits, the study monitors should be trained in the following procedures before embarking on any monitoring visits:

- SOPs regarding the following clinical activities: qualification and selection of PI/clinical site, monitoring of clinical studies, adverse event reporting, and data management to ensure that each person involved in the monitoring process understands his/her role in monitoring the study.
- The monitoring plan of the study, stating the number and frequency of the monitoring visits and what specific tasks are to be done during each visit.

The duties of the study monitor can be summarized as follows:

1. Follow standard operating procedures (SOPs) and the study monitoring plan to ensure that the study is conducted and reported in accordance with the study protocol, applicable regulations, and sponsor SOPs.
2. Review all adverse events and source documents supporting the adverse events.
3. Discuss with the study investigator and the chief medical officer at the sponsor the discovery of any new adverse events, upgrade or downgrade of adverse events to or from SAEs.

4. Be available around the clock for consultation or reporting of serious adverse events.
5. Oversee and report on the progress of the study.
6. Alert the investigator to any protocol deviation that occurred in the study. The investigator must report these deviations on the CRFs and also report these deviations to his/her IRB in accordance with the IRB policy.
7. Keep a written record on the monitoring visit in the visits' log.
8. After completion of the monitoring visit, send a letter to the study investigator listing the major findings and recommending the appropriate course of action to correct deficiencies.
9. If an investigator meeting serves to replace the on-site initiation visit, all the instructions regarding the initiation visit must be addressed during the meeting.

Monitoring Plan

Monitoring involves keeping a detailed plan of the monitoring visits that records information on the number, frequency of monitoring visits, and the duty of the monitor at each visit. A detailed monitoring plan is usually discussed in the clinical protocol and includes the following key points:

- Who will perform monitoring visits
- Type and frequency of monitoring visits (initiations, interim monitoring, close-out)
- Number of interim monitoring visits
- What will be monitored on the visits? CRFs? At what percentage (100% or less)?
- Responsibilities of the study monitors at each study visit

The monitoring plan specifies the type of monitoring visit and what is going to be reviewed at each visit. For example, study initiation visits that are to occur prior to the initiation of patient enrollment, as will be discussed later in this chapter, are conducted to promote training on study product and study protocol, as well as the principles of adverse event definitions/reporting.

The interim monitoring visits are usually scheduled over the span of the study, starting with an early monitoring visit after study patients meet study eligibility criteria and are enrolled in the study. This early visit is conducted to review and correct any deficiencies that may occur during the enrollment period. The rest of the interim monitoring visits are distributed to cover the study follow-up visits.

The study close-out visit is usually planned to review and retrieve all remaining monitored CRFs and complete the final investigational product accountability.

Type of Study Visits and Related Clinical Activities

The study site visits conducted by the sponsor can be grouped into four categories: (1) investigator/site qualification visit, (2) study initiation visit, (3) interim monitoring visits, and (4) study close-out visit.

Investigator/Site Qualification Visit The first visit is performed during the preparation phase for the study. The objective of the visit is to select a qualified investigator and an adequate clinical site for the study.

Study Initiation Visit Prior to initiation of subject enrollment in the study, a visit is conducted to train the investigator and research staff on the investigational device, the clinical protocol procedures, and the principals of GCP. The sponsor clinical representative(s) will present and discuss with the research team at the research site the following topics:

- Clinical protocol
- Device description
- Adverse events
- Monitoring plan
- Case report forms
- Responsibilities of the PI
- Informed consent form
- Protocol deviations

The sponsor representative may give a quiz at the end of the training to ensure that the level of understanding of the PI and his/her research staff is adequate.

Interim Monitoring Visits Visits conducted during the course of patient enrollment and follow-up visits are planned to supervise study procedures (subject enrollment, baseline assessments, study procedures, and follow-up visits). The sponsor's clinical representative reviews and monitors the accuracy of CRFs, adverse events and its supporting source documents, and also documents in the study's regulatory binder. Specifically the interim monitoring visits are designed to achieve the following:

- The investigator has a mechanism by which he/she may identify the treatment of a particular participant.
- The informed consent for each participant has been obtained prior to commencement of any protocol required activity.
- All investigational products are used according to the conditions in the protocol.
- The investigator retains all necessary study documentation.
- Source data are available to ascertain the existence of the participant and enable information recorded in the CRFs.
- Any changes to the CRFs are properly documented, signed, and dated.
- The investigational product(s) are managed in accordance with the protocol.

The monitor conducting the visit as well as any staff of the sponsor present during the visit will sign the Monitoring Visit Log. At a minimum, during these visits the monitor will accomplish the following:

- Review regulatory documents for completeness and accuracy and to ensure that all documents are current, especially IRB/EC reviews and approvals.
- Ensure that all subjects have completed a current and correct version of an Informed Consent (including HIPAA and/or Assent, if appropriate) prior to any study procedures being conducted.
- Ensure that any serious and/or unanticipated device adverse effects are documented and appropriately reported to the sponsor and to the IRB/EC in accordance with the IRB policy.
- Ensure that all AEs are captured in the CRF.
- Assess compliance with the protocol.
- Assess whether recruitment/enrollment meet requirements as specified in the protocol.
- Review source documents and compare them against CRFs to ensure accurate and complete collection of study data and that any appropriate data corrections are completed.

- Review and ensure completion of any outstanding data queries.
- Review outstanding issues with site staff and ensure their resolution or discuss a plan for their resolution.
- Assess compliance of the site with requirements for investigational product use, storage, and accountability.

Each follow-up visit is documented in an Interim Monitoring Visit Report, which is completed by the monitor. The report includes:

- Resolved and outstanding issues
- The progress of the study, determination of recruitment status, number of subject withdrawals; the activities of the principal investigator and the staff and the continuing ability of the center to participate in the study; adherence to the protocol and related documents
- Missing visits or examinations
- Subjects failing to complete the study and the reason for each failure
- Confirmation that informed consent is in accordance with 21 CFR Parts 50 and 56

Study Close-out Visit   The final visit is performed after the last patient in the study completes the last follow-up visit. In this visit the sponsor retrieves all remaining CRFs, and completes all device inventories. In the close-out visit the sponsor should achieve the following:

- Finalize device accountability inventory to ensure that all devices used in the study are accounted for.
- Verify that all patients case report forms are completed and all copies of the case report forms are retrieved from the site.
- Close all open items from previous monitoring visits.
- Complete the site regulatory file review.
- Ensure that complete documentation of all clinical and laboratory investigations is available in the CRFs.
- Ensure that all adverse events are documented and reported appropriately.
- Confirm that the principal investigator has notified the study participants, ethics committees and, if required, regulatory authorities that the study has been completed.

Record of On-site Visits The following information needs to be recorded about each study visit:

- Date of the visit
- Name(s) of individual(s) who conduct the visit
- Name and address of the investigator visited
- Statement of the findings, conclusions, and actions taken to correct any deficiencies noted during the visit

MONITORING REPORTS

Type of Monitoring Report

Study monitoring reports are completed by the sponsor or its designee in accordance with the following types of the monitoring visits:

- PI and site qualification report
- Initiation visit report
- Interim monitor visits reports
- Study close-out report

PI and Site Qualification Report

The principal investigator (PI) and site qualification report includes an evaluation of the PI, research staff, and research facility for the purpose of selecting a research investigator and research facility for the study. This report is covering the following topics:

- Names and titles of site staff evaluated in this visit
- Name and title of sponsor representative conducted this visit
- Facility review
- PI review

Initiation Visit Report

The initiation visit report should include the following items:

- Names and titles of site staff present in this visit
- Name and title of sponsor representative(s) conducting the training

- The training agenda
- Documentation of the training items

Interim Monitoring Visit Report

Interim visit reports should cover the following items:

- Number of patients screened and enrolled in the study
- Findings regarding review of the Study Regulatory Binder
- Findings regarding monitoring of the CRFs
- Review of adverse events CRFs, the discovery of new adverse events that are not reported, or the upgrade or downgrade of adverse events
- Review of any protocol deviations or the discovery of new deviations
- Review of device accountability log

Study Close-out Report

The study close-out visit report includes the following topics:

- Review of final device accountability log
- Ensure that all CRFs are monitored and retrieved
- Confirm that all adverse events are reported appropriately
- Address any unresolved issue(s)

Sample Interim Monitoring Visit Report

The following is an example of the information required for monitoring reports:

Protocol number and version: List the protocol number and version number if applicable.

Protocol title: List the protocol title.

Visit date: Write the visit date.

PI name and address: Write the PI name and address.

Name of monitor and attendees: List the names of the study monitor(s) and attendees at the study site.

Facility review:

- List changes to the study facility since the previous visit.
- Does the site continue to have adequate storage secure place for the study materials and documents?
- Does the site continue to have adequate monitoring area?

Enrollment:

- List the number of subjects enrolled in the study.
- Report if subject enrollment is going in accordance with the plan.

Adverse event reporting: List all adverse events captured and reported accordingly by the study investigator.

Regulatory: Report if study regulatory binder missing any item.

Study findings: Report any action item that the site needs to follow up and complete.

Corrective action: List suggested corrective actions to any of the study findings.

INTERIM MONITORING VISIT REPORT TEMPLATE

Protocol No.	Visit Date(s):	Study Device:
Protocol Name:		
Investigator Name / No.:	Investigator Address:	

Site Staff Present (Names and Titles)	
Sponsor/Sponsor Representatives Present (Names and Titles)	

Screening and Enrollment Information			
Total Planned Enrollment		Total Active	
Number Screened		Total Completed	
Number Screen Failures		Number of Early Terminations	
Total Enrolled		Number of Deaths	

Instructions: Respond to each item on the following pages by checking Y = Yes, N = No, NA = Not applicable, or NE = Not evaluated. Specify details of responses in the comments section.

Subject Accrual		Y	N	NA	NE
1	Is the current enrollment rate adequate to achieve the agreed-upon goal?	☐	☐	☐	☐
2	Do enrolled subjects meet the inclusion/exclusion criteria?	☐	☐	☐	☐
3	Have there been any subjects enrolled or screened since the previous visit?	☐	☐	☐	☐
4	Have there been any deaths, early terminations or completed subjects since the previous visit?	☐	☐	☐	☐

Facilities Review		Y	N	NA	NE
5	Does the site continue to have adequate facilities and equipment to properly conduct the study?	☐	☐	☐	☐
6	If there were changes to facilities and/or equipment, were they inspected and found to be adequate for safe and proper conduct of the study?	☐	☐	☐	☐
7	Is a suitable, secure and dedicated area being utilized for storage of study documents, CRFs, etc.?	☐	☐	☐	☐
8	Is there an adequate supply of study materials (CRFs, etc.)?	☐	☐	☐	☐
9	Do there continue to be adequate monitoring space and facilities available?	☐	☐	☐	☐

Investigator and Staff Review		Y	N	NA	NE
10	Principal investigator was available for the visit.	☐	☐	☐	☐
11	Study staff was available for the visit.	☐	☐	☐	☐
12	Does the PI continue to have adequate staff to properly conduct the study?	☐	☐	☐	☐
13	If there have been any changes to PI or staff since the previous visit, has the appropriate training been completed for the new staff?	☐	☐	☐	☐
14	Has there been any change in delegation of responsibility at this site?	☐	☐	☐	☐
15	Have any site re-training needs been identified during this visit?	☐	☐	☐	☐
16	Is there any change in site contact information (address, phone numbers, etc.) since the previous visit?	☐	☐	☐	☐

Investigational Product (IP) Review		Y	N	NA	NE
17	Was IP accountability completed during this visit?	☐	☐	☐	☐
	(a) If yes, is the site compliant with all accountability requirements?	☐	☐	☐	☐
	(b) If yes, are all IP shipment, receipt, use and destruction records complete, accurate and current?	☐	☐	☐	☐
18	Is the IP being maintained under the required storage conditions (temperature, humidity, etc.)?	☐	☐	☐	☐
19	Is the IP being stored in a secure location with limited accessibility?	☐	☐	☐	☐
20	Are all devices within the expiration period?	☐	☐	☐	☐
21	Have there been any device complaints at this site since the previous visit?	☐	☐	☐	☐
	(a) If yes, has all appropriate documentation been completed and submitted?	☐	☐	☐	☐

Regulatory Review	Y	N	NA	NE
22	Was the Regulatory Binder/File reviewed at this visit? (*If NO, skip to the next section and describe in comments the reason not reviewed.*)	☐	☐	☐	☐
23	Are all regulatory documents current and complete?	☐	☐	☐	☐
24	Are PI and Sub-I CVs current (signed within the previous 12 months)?	☐	☐	☐	☐
25	Are PI and Sub-I medical licenses current?	☐	☐	☐	☐
26	Are all Financial Disclosure Forms properly completed for all required staff members?	☐	☐	☐	☐
27	Are all Lab certifications/licenses and Lab Director licenses present and current?	☐	☐	☐	☐
28	Are all Lab normal ranges present and current?	☐	☐	☐	☐
29	Are copies of all Protocol versions present?	☐	☐	☐	☐
30	Are all versions of the Instructions for Use present?	☐	☐	☐	☐
31	Are all IRB/EC submissions for and approval of all Protocol versions present and accurate?	☐	☐	☐	☐
32	Are all IRB/EC approvals present for subject materials (ICFs, HIPAA [if required], minor assent, patient information sheets, recruitment advertisement, diaries, etc.)	☐	☐	☐	☐
33	Have all required reports been submitted to IRB/EC?	☐	☐	☐	☐
34	Have all safety reports been submitted to the IRB/EC as required?	☐	☐	☐	☐
35	Were all deviations reported to the IRB/EC, as required?	☐	☐	☐	☐
36	Is the IRB/EC membership roster present and complete?	☐	☐	☐	☐
37	Is all site correspondence current and complete?	☐	☐	☐	☐
38	Have any regulatory documents been collected during this visit for submission to the Proteus TMF?	☐	☐	☐	☐

Informed Consent Document Review	Y	N	NA	NE
39	Have all Informed Consents (including associated HIPAA [if required], minor assent, etc.) documents been reviewed for all screened subjects (including enrolled and screen failures)?	☐	☐	☐	☐
40	Have all versions of the ICF, etc., been approved by the IRB/EC?	☐	☐	☐	☐
41	Has the site used appropriate versions of consent documents for all subjects?	☐	☐	☐	☐
42	Have all screened subjects been appropriately consented prior to performing any study-specific procedures?	☐	☐	☐	☐
43	Has the consent process been appropriately documented in the site source documents?	☐	☐	☐	☐

CRF / Data review	Y	N	NA	NE
44	Is source documentation adequate to be able to do a thorough review of study data?	☐	☐	☐	☐
45	Was source documentation reviewed and compared to CRF data entry in accordance with the Monitoring Plan, the protocol and all other associated guidance (including FDA, GCP, and any other regulatory guidance)?	☐	☐	☐	☐
46	Are all Inclusion/Exclusion criteria being adhered to for all new subjects reviewed during this visit?	☐	☐	☐	☐
47	Has the protocol been adhered to for all subjects reviewed during this visit?	☐	☐	☐	☐
48	Are all Core Lab submissions being made appropriately and on time according to the protocol and/or all associated study guidelines?	☐	☐	☐	☐
49	Were all AEs appropriately captured on CRFs?	☐	☐	☐	☐
50	Are CRFs being completed accurately and in accordance with the protocol and any associated CRF completion guidelines?	☐	☐	☐	☐
51	Are data queries being resolved in a timely and appropriate manner?	☐	☐	☐	☐

Interim Visit Findings		Y	N	NA	NE
52	Are there any new action items resulting from this visit? (If Yes, complete New Action Items section.)	☐	☐	☐	☐
53	Are there any outstanding action items remaining open from the previous visit(s)? (If Yes, complete Outstanding Action Items section.)	☐	☐	☐	☐
54	Were any action items resolved since the previous visit? (If Yes, complete Action Items Closed since Previous Visit section.)	☐	☐	☐	☐

Outstanding Action Items			
Category	Date Created	Issue Description	Recommended Action(s)

New Action Items			
Category	Date Created	Issue Description	Recommended Action(s)

Action Items Closed since Previous Visit				
Category	Date Created	Issue Description	Action(s) Taken	Date Closed

4

ADVERSE EVENTS DEFINITIONS AND REPORTING PROCEDURES

Design, Execution, and Management of Medical Device Clinical Trials, by Salah Abdel-aleem
Copyright © 2009 John Wiley & Sons, Inc.

The evaluation of adverse events occurring in a clinical study is considered a vital safety outcome of the study, and identification and reporting of adverse events remains to be one of the most important and challenging aspects of clinical trials. For optimal reporting on adverse events, it is recommended that the sponsor define in advance all the adverse events that are anticipated to occur in the study, and also provide guidelines and examples for adverse event reporting to the study investigators. The sponsor should then try its best to monitor, review, and even adjudicate, if necessary, adverse events that occur in the study. In certain occasions the sponsor may set up specific committees, such as a Data Safety and Montoring Board (DSMB) and a Clinical Event Committee (CEC), as the ultimate authorities to review and decide on certain serious adverse events or major adverse events in the study. This process should help prevent, or at least, minimize bias in reporting adverse events. These committees are created to develop and assign a uniform process for defining and identifying the study adverse events.[9–12]

In the clinical protocol a separate section should be devoted to the definition of adverse events, serious adverse events, and unanticipated adverse device effects in accordance with the FDA and ICH guidelines. Also, in this section, guidance should be given to the investigator on the potential anticipated adverse events, what information needs to be reported about each adverse event, and the timeline for reporting different types of adverse events, as well as to whom they will report these adverse events. The clinical protocol should define what types of adverse events need be reported throughout the follow-up visits after the completion of the research procedure. The statistical analysis plan (SAP) should include detailed procedures for the analysis of adverse events. A definition should be provided for what is considered a device-related adverse event, serious adverse event, unanticipated device adverse effect, and the grading of the severity or strength of adverse events.

In global clinical studies that include international clinical sites, and where the final report of the study is anticipated to be submitted to the FDA and other international regulatory bodies, it is important to reconcile differences in the definition of certain adverse events and their reporting timelines between the US and other international regions.

Adverse events may include, but are not limited to:

- Subjective or objective symptoms spontaneously offered by the patient or subject and/or observed by the physician or medical staff
- Laboratory abnormalities of clinical significance

Disease signs, symptoms, and/or laboratory abnormalities already existing prior to the use of the product are *not* considered adverse experiences *unless* they re-occur after the patient has recovered from the preexisting condition, or represent an exacerbation in intensity or frequency.

ADVERSE EVENT DEFINITIONS

The different categories of adverse events are defined in accordance with the FDA and the ICH guidelines as adverse, serious adverse, anticipated adverse, and unanticipated adverse events.

Adverse Event (AE)   Any undesirable medical event occurring in a research subject in an adverse event, whether or not the event is considered related to the investigational device.

Serious Adverse Event (SAE)   A SAE is defined as an adverse event that results in:

- Death
- Life-threatening condition
- Hospitalization or prolonged hospitalization
- Required intervention to prevent permanent impairment/damage, disability, or permanent damage
- Congenital anomaly/birth defect
- Other serious important medical event

Anticipated Adverse Event   An adverse event that is listed in the clinical protocol or other study-related document has already been identified as a *potential* AE related to the investigational device or procedure being studied.

Unanticipated Adverse Device Effect (UADE)   Any serious adverse effect on health or safety or any life-threatening problem or death caused by, or associated with, a device, is UADE if that effect, problem, or death *was not previously identified in nature, severity or degree of incidence* in the investigational plan or application. A UADE may also be any other unanticipated serious problem associated with a device that relates to the rights, safety, or welfare of subjects. In summary, UADE are serious adverse events, device related and unexpected.

POLICIES, REGULATIONS, AND GUIDELINES REGARDING ADVERSE EVENT REPORTING

Code of Federal Regulations

The following is the list of applicable FDA and international safety and adverse event regulation:

- CFR Title 21 Part 50 Protection of Human Subjects
- CFR Title 21 Part 56 Institutional Review Boards
- CFR Title 21 Part 312 Investigational New Drug Application
- CFR Title 21 Part 812 Investigational Device Exemption

International Conference on Harmonization (ICH) Guidelines

E6 Good Clinical Practice

E2A Clinical Data Management: Definition and standards for expedited reporting

ADVERSE EVENT REPORTING PATHWAY

The pathway for recognizing, identifying, and reporting an adverse event by the clinical site investigator is illustrated in Figure 4.1. This pathway starts with the investigator of that site becoming aware of the

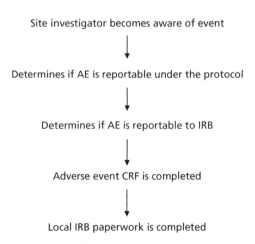

Figure 4.1   Adverse event reporting pathway

occurrence of an adverse event. The investigator checks if this adverse event is reportable under the study protocol (the protocol, the investigator brochure, or instructions for use usually define adverse event categories or list examples of adverse events to be reported in the study). The investigator should report any such adverse events in accordance with his/her IRB policy because certain adverse events that are serious adverse events and/or unanticipated adverse device effects must be reported to the IRB within specified periods of time. Adverse event data should be recorded in the adverse event CRF and the IRB designated forms.

TERMS FOR CAUSALITY ASSESSMENT

The cause–effect relationship between the investigational device, the research procedure, and the investigational device, could be assigned as follows:

Not Related   The experience is clearly related to other factors such as the patient's clinical state, therapeutic intervention, or concomitant therapy.

Unlikely   The experience was probably produced by other factors such as the patient's clinical state, therapeutic intervention, or concomitant therapy, and does not follow a known response pattern to the trial product.

Possible   The experience follows a reasonable temporal sequence from the time of product administration or placement, and/or follows a known response pattern to the trial product, but could have been produced by other factors such as the patient's clinical state, therapeutic intervention, or concomitant therapy.

Most Probable   The experience follows a reasonable temporal sequence from the time of product administration or placement, and/or follows a known response pattern to the trial product, and could not have been produced by other factors such as the patient's clinical state, therapeutic intervention, or concomitant therapy. Further the experience immediately follows the trial product's administration, or improves on stopping the product, or there is positive reaction at the application site.

GAPS/CHALLENGES IN ADVERSE EVENT REPORTING

Several challenges are usually associated with reporting adverse events. Some of these challenges are related to timelines that must be adhered to by site investigators for reporting of serious adverse events or serious unanticipated adverse device effects. Other challenges are associated with the complexity of the study and the level of guidance the sponsor provides for reporting these adverse events.

Challenges of Site Investigators in Adverse Event Reporting

The following challenges may be faced by the principal investigator in reporting adverse events:

- *Definitions of SAE.* If a SAE is identified in the study, source documents should support the designation based on the criteria of SAE. Sometimes it is difficult to determine whether the adverse event is serious or not based on the available source documents.
- *Time frame for reporting.* SAE and serious unanticipated adverse device effects should be reported to the sponsor within the time frame specified by the sponsor for reporting these events. Sometimes the PI becomes aware of certain SAEs after the allowed time period for reporting is passed.
- *Relationship between the event and investigational product.* The investigator should attempt to best define the cause–effect relationship between the study device and the adverse events. Often lack of direct evidence of relationship does present a challenge. This category of events should be further defined as to whether this adverse event is thought to be related or unrelated to the investigational product. An opinion as to the relatedness between the two extremes should be given, such as unlikely to be related, or likely to be related.

Challenges of the Sponsor in Adverse Event Reporting

- *Complete, accurate reporting of the adverse event data, and timeliness of reports.* The sponsor of the study has the obligation to report certain adverse events to the FDA or participating IRB within a specified time frame; therefore the review of all the adverse events must occur before the specified time windows has expired.

• *Determining unexpected events.* The determination of unanticipated adverse effects sometimes become challenging due to study indication or study procedures to be followed.

Adverse Event Recording[9–12]

All adverse events (AEs) must be recorded in the study adverse event case report forms (CRFs). These forms include the following information about an adverse event:

• Description of the AE, including signs and symptoms. Signs of AE include what physicians see (e.g., laboratory tests), whereas symptoms of AE typically refer to how patients describe experiences. AEs are better described when they are based on signs of the disease whenever is possible.
• Whether the AE is a serious adverse event (SAE). If an AE is determined to be a SAE, then the rationale for this determination should be checked.
• Whether the AE is anticipated. Anticipated AEs are usually listed in the study protocol or other study materials (e.g., the instruction for use, IFU) as AEs that can potentially occur in the study.
• Unanticipated AEs. These AEs are likely directly related to the study device.
• Time onset and outcome of AE. Record the start date, stop date, or ongoing documentation if the AE is not completely resolved. In addition the outcome of the adverse event as to whether the event is resolved, not resolved, or resolved with sequelae should be recorded in the adverse event CRFs.
• Relation of the AE to the study device. The relationship of the AE to the study device as to whether the event is related, possibly related, unrelated, or unknown should be recorded in CRFs. Efforts should be devoted to complete this information to the best of the investigators' knowledge, despite the fact that this is often a challenging task.
• Relation of the AE to the study procedure. The relationship of the AE to study procedures as to whether the event is related, possibly related, unrelated, or unknown should be recorded in the adverse event CRFs.
• AE severity. AE severity/intensity should be classified as to whether the AE is mild, moderate, or severe.

- *Mild.* Transient or mild discomfort, no limitation of activity, no medical intervention or therapy required
- *Moderate.* Mild to moderate limitation of activity, some assistance may be needed, no or minimal medical intervention or therapy required
- *Severe.* Marked limitation in activity, some assistance usually needed, medical intervention/therapy/hospitalization required.

ADVERSE EVENT REPORTING TIME PERIODS (21 CFR 803)

- All AEs are reported by the sponsor to IRB/Ethics Committee and the FDA (or other involved regulatory bodies) in the study annual progress reports.
- Serious AEs and serious unanticipated adverse device effects (UADE) must be fully reported by the study investigators to the sponsor within 10 working days of becoming aware of the event.
- The sponsor must fully report to the FDA participating investigators and all reviewing IRB unanticipated adverse device effects within 10 working days of becoming aware of these events.
- The sponsor should terminate the study within 5 days of occurrence of an AE that causes unreasonable safety risks to the study patients.
- UADEs are defined as:
  - AEs that are not identified in study protocol risk analysis
  - AEs that are identified in protocol risk analysis but occur at a rate higher than anticipated
- Studies conducted in the European Union in accordance with EN 540: Severe adverse events and device-related adverse events are reported to the sponsor and reviewing ethics committee. The sponsor reports these adverse events to the relevant authority in 10 days or as required by each EU member state.

DIFFERENCES BETWEEN THE UNITED STATES AND EUROPE IN REPORTING ADVERSE EVENTS

US regulations and the European standard differ in their definition or wording regarding seriousness or severity of an adverse event. The European regulations (EN 540) address adverse event seriousness based on the adverse event severity grading (mild, moderate, severe, and life threatening). The standard explains that a severe adverse event satisfies almost the same condition listed for a serious adverse event in an FDA IDE study (causes death, hospitalization, or prolonged hospitalization; requires intervention; results in a congenital anomaly or malignancy; or results in residual damage. The IDE regulations of the United States use the term *serious* as it is defined above. Many sponsors try to define and describe adverse events based on seriousness as well as severity.

SERIOUS ADVERSE EVENT NARRATIVES

A brief narrative of the SAE is usually completed for each event including the following information:

- Subject gender and age
- Key baseline clinical history items
- Date of the investigational procedure
- Date of the event
- Description of the event
- Whether event is due to the investigational procedure/device
- Event treatment
- Event outcome

Example of Serious Adverse Event Narrative   A 66-year-old female with history of hypertension, peripheral artery disease, myocardial infarction, smoking, and diabetes was admitted to the hospital on 10/1/06, two months after the implantation of the study device, with symptoms of a major stroke. The study procedure was performed on 8/1/06 and the patient was released from the hospital the following day of the procedure without the occurrence of any procedure complications or serious adverse event. The stroke, which occurred two months after the procedure, was confirmed with clinical symptoms and imaging technique (CAT scan). The subject was treated with antithrombolytic therapy for several days in the hospital. The subject was released from the hospital on 10/4/06 with symptoms of paralysis of the left leg, which was confirmed by a CAT scan. Symptoms were confirmed again three months after release from the hospital. This event was judged by the principal investigator and adjudication committee as a serious adverse event, since the adverse event resulted in residual permanent damage. The adverse event was judged by the study PI and the adjudication committee as not related to the study device or procedures.

CLASSIFICATION OF ADVERSE EVENTS

There are several systems available for classification and categorization of adverse events. However, these systems are used differentially in drug and device trails. To best evaluate the safety of an investigational therapy (drug or device), it is helpful to group the adverse events and serious adverse events occurring in the study. One system widely used for classifying adverse events is the System Organ Class–Body System.

WHO SYSTEM ORGAN CLASS–BODY SYSTEM, FOR CLASSIFICATION
OF ADVERSE EVENTS, DRUG SIDE EFFECTS[13]

SOC–ID	SOC–Criteria
01	Infections and infestations
02	Neoplasms benign and malignant (including cysts and polyps)
03	Blood and the lymphatic system disorders
04	Immune system disorders
05	Endocrine disorders
06	Metabolism and nutrition
07	Psychiatric disorders
08	Nervous system disorders
09	Eye disorders
10	Ear and labyrinth disorders
11	Cardiac disorders
12	Vascular disorders
13	Respiratory, thoracic, and mediastinal disorders
14	Gastrointestinal disorders
15	Hepato-biliary disorders
16	Skin and subcutaneous tissue disorders
17	Musculoskeletal, connective tissue and bone disorders
18	Renal and urinary disorders
19	Pregnancy puerperium and prenatal conditions

SOC—ID	SOC—Criteria
20	Reproductive system and breast disorders
21	Congenital and familial/genetic disorders
22	General disorders and administration site conditions
23	Investigations
24	Injury and poisoning
25	Surgical and medical procedures
26	Social circumstances

Analysis of Adverse Events

In evaluating the safety of a study, it is useful to analyze adverse events in accordance with the following time frame of the occurrence of adverse events:

- Device-related adverse events that happen during the placement or attempt at placement of a device, or during the implantation period of the device (device placement-related AE).
- Procedure-related adverse events that correlate with the study research procedures. The time that these adverse events take depends on the procedure's time frame. For example, in surgical clinical trials, procedure-related adverse events may be reported for up to 30 days from the procedure's date.
- Long-term adverse events occur after 30 days (e.g., 3, 6, 9, 12, 24, 36, or 60 months). The reporting of adverse events over the long term follow-up phase of the study is usually with regard to serious or life-threatening events (stroke, myocardial infarction, etc.) and death.

Adverse Event Reporting in Postmarket Studies

A report of adverse events may be required after the market approval of a device. The FDA likes to get an accurate assessment of rare occurring major or serious adverse events such as death, stroke, or myocardial infarction. Post-market studies are usually designed as registries with large sample sizes to get accurate assessments of any major adverse events.

SPECIAL REQUIREMENTS FOR REPORTING CERTAIN ADVERSE EVENTS

The sponsor of the study may determine, prior to initiating the study, that certain serious adverse events or major adverse events (e.g., death, stroke, myocardial infarction) will be judged by a clinical event committee, and this committee will be the ultimate deciding authority on any adverse event. This process minimizes bias in determining adverse events because of the use of a uniform process across study sites.

CASE EXAMPLE

The sponsor became aware of a safety issue that could present a reasonable health risk to a subject at one of the study sites. What should the sponsor do?

- Schedule a meeting as soon as possible with the study PI and his/her research team?
- Discuss in detail the safety concerns:
  - Whether the event presents safety concern to the study subjects
  - Whether the event is related to the investigational product
  - Whether the event is unanticipated
- If the medical reviewer (the sponsor, the investigator, or the DSMB) determines that the event causes serious safety concerns or issues to the study subjects, then the sponsor must stop the research, within an appropriate allowable regulatory time window, until this safety issue is resolved
- The sponsor must communicate this decision to the FDA, other involved regulatory agencies, and all participating IRBs

MANDATORY DEVICE REPORTING FOR FDA-APPROVED DEVICES[14]

User-facilities such as hospitals and nursing homes are legally required to report suspected medical device-related deaths to both FDA and the manufacturer, if known, and serious injuries to the manufacturer or to FDA, if the manufacturer is unknown. These reports must be made on the MedWatch 3500A Mandatory Reporting Form. The instructions for completing the MedWatch 3500A reporting form can be obtained from http://www.fda.gov/cdrh/mdruf.pdf.

5

STATISTICAL ANALYSIS PLAN (SAP) AND BIOSTATISTICS IN CLINICAL RESEARCH

Design, Execution, and Management of Medical Device Clinical Trials,
by Salah Abdel-aleem
Copyright © 2009 John Wiley & Sons, Inc.

This chapter presents an outline of the Statistical Analysis Plan (SAP) along with some basics statistical methods for clinical trials such as determination of the sample size and study hypothesis. After reviewing this chapter, the reader will be familiar with simple statistics terms used for clinical trials such as the requirements for sample size determination, the selection of the study endpoints, the level of clinical and statistical significance of the data. However, it should be noted that this chapter is not intended to provide detailed statistics methods or statistical analysis procedures.

STATISTICAL ANALYSIS PLAN (SAP)

The statistical analysis plan (SAP) refers to the procedures followed by the sponsor of the study to define and analyze the study's endpoints, measurements, and also to provide a basis for the sample size determination of the study. The detailed SAP includes a plan for how the data of the study is to be presented in tables, figures, and listings. In certain FDA-sponsored studies, such as IDE studies, it is useful to discuss the key elements of the SAP with the FDA prior to initiation or during the early stages of the study so that there will be no confusion about such issues between the FDA and the sponsor.

Overview of SAP

The SAP is specifically designed to achieve the following objectives:

- Define and discuss the study hypothesis and how the sample size of the study is determined
- Define and discuss the primary, secondary, and other endpoints of the study
- Set up the study success criteria
- Discuss how the data are going to be presented in the final study report

SAP Contents

The SAP of a clinical study includes the following sections:

1. Introduction
2. Study design and objectives

3. General analysis definitions
4. Demographics and baseline characteristics
5. Patient disposition
6. Investigational product accountability
7. Concomitant therapy
8. Effectiveness analyses
9. Safety analyses
10. Quality of life
11. Economic outcome
12. Pharmacokinetics for some combination products
13. Interim analyses and safety monitoring analyses
14. Protocol violations
15. References

Outline of SAP

The following is a template of the contents of an SAP of a clinical study:

- Introduction
- Study design and objectives
  - Study objectives
      Primary objectives
      Secondary objectives
      Other objectives
  - Trial design
  - Sample size determination
- General analysis definitions
  - Study period and visit window definitions
      Study periods
      Visit windows
  - Study populations
      Intent-to-treat population
      Per-protocol population
      Safety population
      Other populations
  - Subgroup definitions and analysis
  - Treatment assignment and treatment groups

- Center pooling method
- Missing data analysis

As mentioned above, study design, primary, secondary, and other endpoints are discussed in the SAP in accordance with the study protocol. The scientific method used to calculate the study sample size and its justification is also discussed in the SAP. Study population analyses, such as per-protocol population and intent-to-treat population, are defined in the SAP. Definitions of particular subgroups, methods of treatment assignment, data pooling from clinical study centers, and missing data analysis are discussed in detail in the SAP.

Characteristics of SAP for Clinical Trials

THE SAP should have the following characteristics and should provide the following information regarding a given clinical trials:

- A detailed description of the primary and secondary endpoints and how they are to be measured.
- Details of the statistical methods and tests that will be used to analyze the endpoints. The analysis of the primary outcome must follow the principle of intention to treat section.
- The strategy to be used (e.g., alternative statistical procedures) if the distributional or test assumptions are not satisfied.
- Comparisons that may be one-tailed or two-tailed (with appropriate justification if necessary) and the level of significance to be used.
- Any adjustment, as needed, to the significance level or the final P values that will be made to account for any planned or unplanned multiple testing or subgroup analyses.
- Potential adjusted analyses, with a statement of which covariates or factors will be included.
- Any planned subgroup or subset analysis along with justification for the relevance of this analysis (e.g., biological rationale) before commencement of the trial.
- The planned exploratory analyses, justifying their importance.
- Support for differential subgroup effects along with biological rationale and supporting evidence from within and outside the study, as well as statistical evidence of interaction between the overall treatment effect and that observed in the subgroup(s) of interest.

- Any pre-specified subgroups that have more interpretive value than those defined on an ad-hoc basis or as a result of multiple comparisons.

Requirements Regarding SAP

- The SAP is a clearly defined section within the protocol so it must be approved prior to the start of clinical research study.
- The SAP should include the details of the statistical analyses associated with a clinical study. The analyses are planned with the desired work product(s) in mind and should be conducted in a consistent and repeatable manner.
- The SAP should contain the detailed requirements and parameters for the reporting results of the clinical research trial, the format and content of output reports, and the tests to support the robustness and sensitivity of the analysis conducted.
- Recommended checks and specific procedures whose implementation and completion will improve/ensure the quality of the plan and the associated data, as well as prevent the study's compromise, should be included.
- The SAP should include, at a minimum, for each primary and secondary endpoint:
  - How the outcome will be measured.
  - Any transformations on the data likely to be required before analysis.
  - Appropriate statistical tests that will be used to analyze the data.
  - How missing data will be accounted for in the analyses (both scientifically and statistically).
  - Whether statistical inference will be drawn and if any statistical adjustments for multiple comparisons will be performed.

SELECTION OF STUDY ENDPOINTS

- The primary and secondary endpoints of a clinical study are best selected when they are based on previously published clinical studies, or relevant preclinical data
- The study sample size should be designed to prove the primary safety and effectiveness of the endpoint(s)

Primary Effectiveness (Efficacy) Endpoints   The primary effectiveness endpoint should demonstrate the clinical outcome of the therapy such as reduction of mortality and reduction or improvement of hypertension. The magnitude of the clinical significant effect should be determined, and this is best selected when it is objectively measured.

Primary Safety Endpoints   This endpoint determines the rates of certain major adverse events in a particular study, primarily death, but also stroke or MI, to assess the safety of the product.

Secondary Endpoints   Secondary endpoints are designed to achieve the following:

- These endpoints are usually designed to evaluate the rate of certain adverse events, to capture procedure complications, rate of device failures, and technical success or performance of certain parameters of a device.
- The validity of certain effectiveness endpoints is tested because clinical studies are not usually powered enough to prove the study secondary endpoints that support the primary endpoint of the study and also test the utility of these endpoints for future studies.

Selection of Hard and Soft Endpoints

Endpoints
- Desirable features of endpoints
  - Relevant to disease process, easy to interpret
  - Free from measurement or assessment error
  - Sensitive to treatment differences
  - Measurable within a reasonable period of time

"Hard" Endpoints
- Quantitative measurements of hard endpoints:
  - Well-defined in study protocol
  - Definitive with respect to disease process
  - Not subjective
- Examples:
  - Death
  - Time to disease progression/relapse
  - Some laboratory measurements

"Soft" Endpoints   Soft endpoints are not directly related to disease process or require subjective assessment by patient/physician. Examples are quality of life questionnaires and symptom questionnaires.

Surrogate Endpoints[15,16]

In certain studies it is difficult to determine the clinical outcome such as mortality or survival due to increased study sample size and other factors. In these situations surrogate endpoints may be used as primary endpoints of the study to reduce the cost and duration of the study. Surrogate endpoints are measurable endpoints that are directly related to the clinical outcome of the study, such as effect of antidiabetic therapies on the blood sugar level or antihypertensive therapies on blood pressure. For a surrogate endpoint to be an effective substitute for the clinical outcome, effects of the intervention on the surrogate must reliably predict the overall effect on the clinical outcome. However, in practice, this could fail because of the possibility that the disease process could affect the clinical outcome through several causal pathways that are not mediated through the surrogate. The intervention effect on these pathways would then be different from the effect on the surrogate; see Figure 5.1.

Several causal pathways of the disease could affect the clinical outcome without affecting the surrogate. Also the surrogate is not in the pathway of the intervention effect.

The meta-analysis study performed by Gordon[17] on the effect of lipid-lowering agents on mortality showed no correlation between lowering lipids and mortality; as a matter of fact mortality was increased by 1% in response to lipid-lowering agents in these studies. In contrast, evidence has been established for the relationship between lowering hypertension and reducing mortality or stroke.[18]

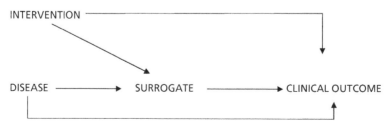

Figure 5.1   Effects of disease and intervention on surrogate endpoint and clinical outcome

Composite Endpoints[19,20]

Composite endpoints are commonly used in randomized controlled clinical trials because they offer potential advantages, such as smaller sample sizes and shorter duration of the study. A composite endpoint in a RCT consists of multiple single endpoints that are combined in order to confront an investigational treatment with a higher number of events expected during the trial. For instance, the primary composite endpoint may include mortality along with nonfatal endpoints such as hospitalization and cardiac arrest in chronic heart failure patients, or along with myocardial infarction and stroke in hypertensives. The major advantages in using a composite endpoint are statistical precision and efficiency can be increased, trials become smaller and less costly, and the results of promising new treatments become available earlier. If more than one outcome is important for efficacy evaluation, a composite endpoint can efficiently deal with the issue of multiplicity.

Requirements of the Composite Endpoints   The use of a composite endpoint in a clinical trial usually has the following requirements:

- The individual components of the composite are clinically meaningful and of similar importance to the patient.
- The expected effects on each component are similar, based on biological plausibility.
- The clinically more important components of composite endpoints should at least not be affected negatively.

Disadvantage of Composite Endpoints
- The selected individual components of a composite endpoint are not always clinically meaningful.
- The problems with nonvalidated surrogate endpoints need to be kept in mind when selecting outcome variables for the composite, particularly when a relationship between the surrogate and mortality has not been established.
- A "worst-case scenario" happened in the CAPRICORN trial, which investigated carvedilol in patients with left-ventricular dysfunction after myocardial infarction. The original endpoint, all-cause mortality, was changed during the trial to a new composite consisting of mortality and hospital admissions. Whereas the "old" endpoint achieved a P value of 0.03, the "new" combined endpoint, in contrast, failed to show statistical significance.

Changing the Primary Outcome during the Conduct of the Study

Circumstances can arise where, after a trial commences, the primary outcome is deemed to be suboptimal. This most commonly occurs when the observed rate of the primary outcome is substantially lower than anticipated, reducing the ability (power) of the study to evaluate the effects of treatment on this outcome. This could be the result of a recent change in nontrial background therapy or to recruitment of a healthier subset of the patients of interest. In these instances it is possible to modify the primary outcome, provided that the reason for doing so *is not based on knowledge of interim results of the effect of treatment in the study*. Thus, if study data indicate that the rate of myocardial infarction (the primary outcome) is much lower in the intervention or control arm than originally anticipated, it would be highly inappropriate to modify the primary outcome to, for example, include stroke, as this choice is potentially influenced by a knowledge of interim results of the effects of treatment in the study. However, using the overall event rate for myocardial infarction in the whole study cohort (blinded—not differentiated by treatment) could provide justification for endpoint modification in a valid way. Any change in primary outcome during the study requires careful thought, planning, and documentation.

BIOSTATISTICS IN CLINICAL RESEARCH

Study Hypothesis

- A clear hypothesis is normally designed for the study
- The hypothesis should be stated in terms of clinical significance (e.g., reduction of mortality by 10%)

Hypothesis Testing

- The objective of statistics is usually to make inferences about unknown population parameters based on information contained in a sample. These inferences can be phrased in one of two ways:
  - Estimates of the parameters
  - Tests of hypotheses about their values
- Statistics are useful in assisting with:
  - How to decide when to accept or reject a hypothesis?
  - What is the probability that a wrong decision is made?
  - What function of the sample measurements should be used to make this decision?

Null Hypothesis $(\mathbf{H_0})$[21]
  - The sponsor generally develops a theory or research hypothesis to be tested.
  - In a clinical trial two treatments are compared, the null hypothesis is "no difference between treatments"

$$H_0 : \text{Treatment A} = \text{Treatment B}$$

  - If the means of two populations are compared, μ1 & μ2, for equality, the null hypothesis is "the means are equal".

$$H_0 : \mu_1 = \mu_2$$

Type I and II Errors
  - A type I error (known as α) in statistical tests describes the chance of rejecting the null hypothesis when it is in fact true. The value of α is usually set to 0.05.
  - A type II error (Known as β) reflects the conclusion that there is no evidence that a treatment works when it actually does work. In statistical tests β describes the chance of not rejecting the null hypothesis when it is in fact false. The value of β is usually set up at 0.2.

Power   The power of a hypothesis is one minus the probability of type II error $(1 - \beta)$. In clinical trials power is the probability that a trial will detect, as statistically significant, an intervention effect of a specified size. If a clinical trial had a power of 0.8 (or 80%), and assuming that the prespecified treatment effect truly existed, then if the trial was repeated 100 times, it would find a statistically significant effect in 80 of them. Ideally we want a test to have a high power, close to maximum of one (or 100%). The FDA standard is to accept clinical trials with at least 80% power.

One must keep in mind that subjects missing primary endpoint data may decrease the pre-set value for the power of the study. The power should be set high enough initially to account for such occurrences. Often these issues are resolved by attempting to anticipate addition of more subjects than that calculated in the pre-determined sample size to compensate for patients who miss the primary endpoint evaluation, withdrew consent, or were lost to follow-up.

Calculating Sample Sizes[22,23]

The sample size of the study can be predicted if the following parameters are known:

- The significance level α (α is set at 0.05)
- The value of β, since the power is defined as $1 - \beta$, and the power is set up at least at 80% for a pivotal clinical trial.
- The size of the difference to be detected, which is usually determined by what is clinically meaningful (e.g., 10% reduction in mortality rate). This is usually derived from previous clinical studies, previous publications, or the opinion of the key thought leader in the field of research.
- The variance of the data in the samples (mean $\pm$ SD). This is usually derived from previous clinical studies, or previous publications to get a sense of acceptable or normal variation in such measurements.

The sample size of the study can be decreased by:

- Allowing for a bigger type I error
- Allowing for a bigger type II error
- Increasing the level of improvement one expects to achieve
- Choosing a more powerful way of testing
- For a binary endpoint, choosing the one that is closest to 50% in likelihood of being observed in the control arm
- For survival endpoints, extending the length of follow-up
- For continuous measures, decreasing the variation in the outcome

Example of the Study Hypothesis

The study hypothesis will be explained by way of the following example. Say that the research question is: For some disease A, is the mean value of a critical outcome variable, greater for the device-treated group than for the control group?

Two hypotheses would be formulated: *a null hypothesis* that states that the mean value of patients post treatment in the treatment group is equal to (or worse than) that in the controls; and an alternative (or research) hypothesis that states that the mean value post treatment in the treatment group is greater than that in the controls. There are two types of decision errors that can be made by inferring results from a sample to the population. If the sample indicates that the mean is greater in the device-treated group than in the controls (i.e., rejecting the null hypothesis) when in the population there is no difference between means, a *type I error* (α) is made. If, on the other hand, the sample indicates no difference between means, (i.e., accepting the null hypothesis) when the device mean is actually greater, then a *type II error* is made. The probability of making a type II error (β) and statistical power is defined as $1 - \beta$.

The probabilities of these two types of errors occurring rely heavily on sample size calculations for the hypothesis tests. Usually these probabilities are fixed in advance, giving more weight to the error with the more serious consequences. For example, a type I error occurs if the aim of the trial is to show that the test device is "better than" the control, and we falsely reject the null hypothesis, and conclude that the device may be better than the comparison device, when in fact it is equivalent or even worse than the control. Conversely, if the objective of the trial is to show that the device mean survival is "as good as" (really, "no worse than") that of the control, then it would be more serious to accept a false null hypothesis (a type II error). Additionally clinical trial hypothesis tests should involve clinically meaningful differences, that is, those differences in the outcome variable(s) determined by experts in the medical community to be clinically significant. The most common sample size formulas include an estimate of the variability of the clinically meaningful difference in the numerator and an estimate of the clinically meaningful difference to be detected in the denominator. Thus, for a given outcome variable, the larger the variability, the larger the sample size that will be required. Similarly, for a given variability, the smaller the clinical difference to be detected, the larger the sample size.

Basis for Justification of Statistical Procedures[24]

The following statistical tests are used to justify data outcome:

- *t-Test (paired and unpaired).* A statistical hypothesis test used to compare continuous data in two groups and derived from the "*t*" distribution (also called *Student's t-test*).
- *ANOVA.* An analysis of the variation present in an experiment. It is a test of the hypothesis that the variation in an experiment is no greater than that due to normal variation of individuals' characteristics and error in their measurement.

- *Correlation and regression.* A measure of association between two variables. The variables are not designated as dependent or independent.
- *Chi-squared test.* A statistical test based on comparison of a test statistic to a chi-squared distribution. Used in RevMan analyses to test the statistical significance of the heterogeneity statistic.
- *Fisher's exact test.* A statistical significance test used in the analysis of categorical data where sample sizes are small.
- *Choice of* α *(0.05) and* β *(0.2).*
- *P Value.* The probability (ranging from zero to one) that the results observed in a study (or results more extreme) could have occurred by chance if in reality the null hypothesis were true.
- *Statistical significance difference between groups*:
  - $P < 0.05$
  - $P < 0.01^*$
  - $P < 0.001^{**}$
  - $P < 0.0001^{***}$
  - $P < 0.05$ is statistically significant, $P < 0.01, 0.001, 0.0001$ are highly significant
- *95% Confidence intervals for parameter estimates.* A measure of the uncertainty around the main finding of a statistical analysis. Estimates of unknown quantities, such as the *odds ratio* comparing an experimental intervention with a control, are usually presented as a point estimate and a 95% confidence interval. This *means* that if someone were to keep repeating a study in other samples from the same population, 95% of the confidence intervals from those studies would contain the true value of the unknown quantity. Alternatives to 95%, such as 90% and 99% confidence intervals, are sometimes used. Wider intervals indicate lower precision; narrow intervals, greater precision.

Difference between Clinical Statistics and Clinical Practice

Statistical Significance   The influence of chance on the outcome are reflected by the *P* values $< 0.05, 0.01, 0.001,$ and 0.0001.

Clinical Significance   The medical value of the outcome is reflected in small differences between large groups, which can be statistically significant but clinically meaningless. For example, the fasting blood glucose between two groups shows the blood glucose to be 75 mg/dl in one group and 95 mg/dl in the other group. The difference between the two groups could be statistically significant; however, this difference is clinically meaningless because the level of blood glucose in either group is within the normal fasting blood glucose level.

A Priori and A Posteriori Hypotheses

An a priori hypothesis can be proved or disproved by the designed study, whereas an a posteriori hypothesis can provide this outcome but generate new ideas to be proved or disproved in a future study.

Measurement Scales—Discrete or Continuous Scales

Discrete Scale   Whole units are used that are not subdivided.

Frequencies: number of patients with symptoms (independent events)
Counts: number of episodes (not independent events)

Continuous Scale   Numbers used cover a range of amounts that are subdividable, such as body temperature and blood pressure.

Bases of Comparison between Study Groups

The following parameters are used to compare study groups:

- Differences between means, proportions, and odd ratios
- Change from baseline
- Ratio of the means
- Percentage of change
- Percentage of change over time
- Rate of occurrence
- Time until occurrence

Study Outcome

Primary Outcome   Most important dependent variables (endpoints) relate to the study's hypothesis, so they constitute the basis for the sample size calculation.

Secondary Hypothesis   Other measurements of interest may relate to the study's hypothesis.

Minimization of Bias in Clinical Trials

Certain procedures or precautions should be undertaken to prevent, or at least minimize, bias in clinical trials:

- Standardize outcome assessments and the use of objective endpoints. The use of objective study primary endpoint(s) is one of the best ways to avoid a data evaluator bias.
- Eliminate different interpretations of the test reports by selecting an independent study core laboratory for the entire study. Selection of the core laboratory for evaluation of the imaging tests in a particular study should be to minimize bias.
- Randomization of subjects participating in the study into control and experimental arms is important for achieving equivalent groups and the distribution of any confounder baseline characteristics among the groups.
- Double blinding, where both the participating subject and the treating physician are blinded to treatment, is a very effective way to eliminate bias in a trial.
- Special study committees such as DSMB or CEC can be set up. Other special study committees such as the data safety and monitoring board (DSMB) and clinical event adjudication committee (CEC) should also use uniform criteria during the course of the study to define serious and major adverse events in the study.

Economic Evaluation and Clinical Decision Making[25]

The ultimate objective of economic evaluation is to provide a menu of choices for decision making. To do this, the analysis has to include the health costs and outcomes of at least two alternatives, or else the evaluation will be only partial and incomplete.

Defining Health Economic Outcomes

- In the context of health economics, the term[11] outcomes[11] refers to the results of medical interventions and encompasses both cost outcomes and health outcomes.
- Cost outcomes refer to the economic consequences of choosing a particular therapeutic approach.
- Health outcomes include traditional clinical endpoints (e.g., blood pressure, metabolic rate, serum cholesterol).
- Patient-centered outcomes relate to health-related quality of life questionnaire (e.g., functional status, wellness status).

Examples of Cardiac Outcome Measures   The following are examples of the cardiac outcome measurements in clinical trials:

- Symptoms reduced
- Length of stay reduced
- Myocardial infarction avoided
- Lives saved
- Life-years gained
- Quality-adjusted life-years gained (QALYs)

Clinical Outcomes
- Absolute risk reduction (ARR) is the difference in the event rate between control group (C) and treated group (T):

$$ARR = C - T * 100$$

- Relative risk reduction (RRR) is the percentage reduction in events in the treated group event rate (T) compared to the control group event rate (C):

$$RRR = \frac{(C - T)}{C * 100}$$

- Number needed to treat (NNT) is the number of patients who need to be treated to prevent one bad outcome. It is the inverse of the ARR:

$$NNT = \frac{100}{ARR}$$ (use 100 since we're talking in %)

Types of Economic Evaluations

Cost-Minimization Analysis   Cost minimization analysis is used to assess cost differences, where the clinical effectiveness of two alternatives is found to be equal.

Cost-Effectiveness Analysis   Clinical effects are assessed in terms of the costs for some additional health gain (e.g., cost per additional MI prevented).

Cost-Utility Analysis   Clinical outcomes (health states) are converted into utility scores such as the SF-36 or the EuroQol (EQ-5D) in order to estimate quality-adjusted life-years (QALYs).

Cost-Benefit Analysis   This analysis converts different clinical effects into monetary terms as costs and compares the costs.

Bayesian Statistics[26,27]

An approach to statistics based on application of Bayes's theorem that can be used in a single study or meta-analysis. The Bayes theorem relates the conditional and marginal probabilities of two random events. It is often used to compute postain probabilities given observations. A Bayesian analysis uses Bayes's theorem to transform a prior distribution for an unknown quantity (e.g., an odds ratio) into a posterior distribution for the same quantity, in light of the results of a study or studies. The prior distribution may be based on external evidence, common sense, or subjective opinion. Statistical inferences are made by extracting information from the posterior distribution, and these may be presented as point estimates, and credible intervals (the Bayesian equivalent of confidence intervals). The advantages of using the Bayesian statistics include (1) providing direct probability statements, (2) formally incorporating previous information in statistical inference of a data set, and (3) allowing multiple looks at accumulating study data by way of flexible, adaptive research designs. The primary disadvantage is the element of subjectivity, which some think is not scientific. The FDA[27] has developed some guidance for the use of Bayesian statistics, indicating that when good prior information is available for a medical device, for example, from earlier studies on previous generations of the device or from studies overseas, these studies can often be used as prior information because the mechanism of action of medical devices is typically physical, making the effects local and not systemic. Local effects are often predictable from prior information when modifications to a device are minor.

One Important application for the use of Bayesian statistics is the "adaptive sample size" approach of new proposed studies based on data available from previously conducted studies or interim analysis of certain studies. An example of this process may include the existence of data at a certain time interval (12 months) and the need to predict the sample if this study is continued for 24 months. The following information is needed from prior data to predict the sample size at 24 months: the % success rate of the control and treatment, the noninferiority margin, the type I error (which is usually set at 0.05), and the power of the study (which is usually set at a minimum of 0.80). The interim analysis data, or the a priori, should be adequately powered and any incomplete data should be imputed. Also simulated trials where the study success is obtained should consider the examination of the transition probability and model extremes. Using the example of data available from 12 month analysis to predict the sample size at 24 month, data transition probability at 3 to 6 and to 12 month should be examined. The adaptive sample size approach could be used to predict the sample size for a confirmatory trial after only one subgroup showed significant outcome in a previous study. One potential problem is that the prior subgroup original trial may be biased due to "fishing" for a significant subgroup. One solution of this may include results from other subgroups in a hierarchical model. Other challenges and difficulties may include the need of the same requirements of good trial design, and extensive pre-planning including selecting and adjusting prior information.

Meta-analysis Studies[28–32]

Meta-Analysis   A statistical analysis that combines or integrates the results of several independent clinical trialsis considered a meta-analysis. Combined analyses may be applicable to collections of research that are empirical, rather than theoretical; produce quantitative results, rather than qualitative findings; examine the same constructs and relationships; have findings that can be configured in a comparable statistical form (as effect sizes, correlation coefficients, odds ratios, etc.)

Strengths of Meta-Analysis
- Imposes a discipline on the process of summing up research findings
- Represents findings in a more differentiated and sophisticated manner than conventional reviews
- Is capable of finding relationships across studies that are obscured in other approaches
- Protects against overinterpreting differences across studies
- Can handle large numbers of studies (this would overwhelm traditional approaches to review)

Weaknesses of Meta-Analysis
- Requires a good deal of effort

- Mechanical aspects don't lend themselves to capturing more qualitative distinctions between studies
- "Apples and oranges"; comparability of studies is often in the "eye of the beholder"
- Selection bias poses continual threat of neglecting negative and null finding studies that the clinical investigator was unable to find and also outcomes for which there were negative or null findings that were not reported

Pooling of Trial Results-Confounders It should be noted that studies used for meta-analysis should be similar despite the fact that they are not identical. Also not all studies in the pool are placebo-controlled. The conclusions drawn from pooled trial results have to be interpreted with great caution.

Kaplan–Meier Survival Curves[33]

After a clinical trial is executed, there is a follow-up period. During the follow-up the scientists attempt to determine whether the proposed treatment was successful. One of the most common measures in clinical trials is death.

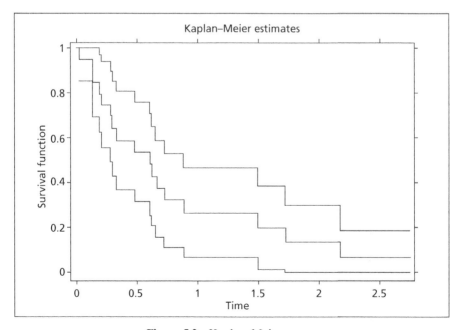

Figure 5.2 Kaplan–Meier curves

However, patients involved in trials do not always complete the follow-up, thus creating data that are not fully accurate. For example, if the follow-up period is 12 years, patients may actually leave after 4 years. A patient that does this frustrates the trial as a result, as the pre-described time frame cannot be concluded. Thus the Kaplan–Meier estimation for survival curves attempts to provide the researchers with a viable interpretation of the data.

An important advantage of the Kaplan–Meier curve is that the method can take into account "censored" data—losses from the sample before the final outcome is observed (e.g., if a patient withdraws from a study). On the plot, small vertical tick-marks indicate losses, where patient data have been censored. When no truncation or censoring occurs, the Kaplan–Meier curve is equivalent to the empirical distribution. Kaplan–Meier survival curves usually draw the correlation between survival and time. The Kaplan–Meier survival curves look like those presented in Figure 5.2.

6

FINAL CLINICAL STUDY REPORT

The final clinical study report is the document that includes the final data of the clinical study and a thorough preparation of this document should be done before submitting the report to regulatory authorities. The approval of the investigational product for marketing or allowing study to proceed to the next phase is largely dependent on the integrity and success of data presented in the report.

Design, Execution, and Management of Medical Device Clinical Trials,
by Salah Abdel-aleem
Copyright © 2009 John Wiley & Sons, Inc.

The clinical report consists of several sections, including an administrative section on the procedures and methodology used throughout the study to ensure the quality and integrity of the data. The administrative sections in the report consist of a protocol synopsis (i.e., a summary of purpose, objectives, design, and the SAP of the study), a description of the precise methodology or procedures followed in the study (e.g., at the core laboratory, core imaging testing centers), and the names of the study committees (e.g., DSMB, Event Adjudication Committee). The other sections of the final report include discussions of the study data analyses (e.g., analyses of demographic and baseline characteristics, the safety and effectiveness analysis, the analysis of adverse events, and the subgroup analysis).

The success of any final study report submitted to the FDA depends on meeting all of the study's primary endpoints and having few compliance issues that raise concern regarding the data integrity of the study. Therefore an account of certain compliance issues, such as missing study follow-up visits, any missing data analysis and its impact on the study's outcome, should be included in the report.

After completing the final study report, It is always prudent to review this document thoroughly to ensure that there are no inconsistencies from section to section in this document.

FINAL CLINICAL REPORT'S OUTLINE

- Executive Summary
- Protocol Synopsis
  - Purpose of the Study
  - Indication
  - Study Design
    - An Overview
    - Inclusion/Exclusion Criteria
    - Study Endpoints
    - Study Experimental Procedures
    - Patients' Follow-up Visits
- Study Centers and Patient Enrollment per Each Study Center: List of all study centers (plus the name and address of the PI at the study center) and the number of patients enrolled per each center.
- Patients' Baseline Characteristics
  - Demographic
    - Age (value ± SD)

- Gender (% male per total participants)
- Race (% of patients)
  - White
  - Black
  - American Indian
  - Hispanic
  - Asian
  - Other
- Weight (value in Ibs ± SD)
- Height (value in inches ± SD)
- Past Medical and Surgical History
  - Physical Exam
  - Concomitant Medications
- Patients Who Met Inclusion/Exclusion Criteria: A list of patients who met the study inclusion/exclusion criteria.
- Patients' Who Did Not Meet Inclusion/Exclusion Criteria and the Reasons for Not Meeting These Criteria: A list of the inclusion/exclusion criteria that were not met and the number of patients who did not meet each criteria.
- Investigational Device Accountability
  - Number of Devices Received
  - Number of Devices Used
  - Number of Devices Returned
- Device Malfunctions/Issues/Problems: A list of all device malfunctions, failures, and the issues surrounding these occurrences (description of the malfunction event, explanation of whether this event affected study data or resulted in adverse events, and discussion of how this malfunction event was resolved: e.g., the device was replaced).
- Study Objectives
  - Primary Objectives
    - Definition of Parameters
    - Definition of Success Criteria
    - Discussion of Whether the Primary Objective Was Met
  - Secondary Objectives
    - Definition of Parameters
    - Definition of Success
    - Discussion of the Results of the Secondary Endpoints

- Safety Evaluations
  - Number of Patients with Adverse Events, Serious Adverse Events, Device-Related Adverse Events, and Procedure-Related AEs: The list is categorized in accordance with the body system.
  - Adverse Event Severity: The number of AEs classified as mild, moderate, and severe in the study.
  - Adverse Events Narratives
  - Description and Classification of AEs
  - Adverse Event Severity/Intensity
  - Device and Procedure-Related AEs
  - Device Malfunction/Performance Issues That Resulted in Adverse Events
- Study Compliance Analysis
  - Number of Patients Completing the Study
  - Number of Patients Missing Follow-up Visits
  - Number of Patients with Compliance Issues
  - Number of Protocol Deviations
  - Type of Protocol Deviations
    - Number of Patients with Inclusion/Exclusion Criteria Deviations
    - Number of Patients with Procedure Protocol Deviations
    - Number of Patients with Compliance Deviations
- Multivariate Analysis
- Examination of Data across Study Sites
- Subgroup Analysis
  - Demographic
  - Study Endpoints
  - Safety Evaluations
- Missing Data Analysis
  - Missing Data That Affected Primary and Secondary Endpoints
  - Missing Data That Affected Study Compliance
- Study Conclusions

DISCUSSION OF SECTIONS IN THE FINAL CLINICAL REPORT

Executive Summary

The executive summary presents the key findings in the study, such as the number of subjects and sites participating in the study, the primary and secondary endpoints. A summary of all safety issues is included as well as of adverse events and serious/major adverse events. The executive summary may further include conclusions and recommendations for the study.

Summary of Methodology and Procedures Followed in the Study

The next section of the report provides a protocol synopsis that includes the purpose, indication for use, patient inclusion/exclusion criteria, endpoints, experimental procedures, and patients' follow-up visits. Additionally this section documents any special procedures followed or study committees set up to prevent or at least limit bias in analyzing the data (e.g., DSMB, CEC, steering committee, or core laboratories used in the study). Also included are a discussion of the study's endpoints and a definition of patient and study success.

Study Centers and Patient Enrollment in Each Study Center— "Patient Disposal or Accountability"

All study centers are listed along with names and addresses of the PIs at the study centers and the number of patients enrolled per each center. Check for inconsistencies regarding patients' enrollment, such as patients enrolled twice by mistake and clinical sites that were activated but did not enroll any patients. This section should cover in more detail the number of patients who did not meet certain inclusion/exclusion criteria, and the criteria not met should be noted.

Analysis of Patients' Baseline Characteristics

Baseline demographic characteristics such as age, gender, race, weight, height, past medical and surgical histories, physical exams, and concomitant medications are discussed in this section and augmented by a statistical presentation of the data (average $\pm$ SD, low and high range, percentage of patients out of the total population, etc.). At the end of this section a summary of the patients who met study inclusion/exclusion criteria and the patients who did not meet the criteria is provided; the reasons for not meeting the criteria are also given in this section. It should be noted that the total number of subjects available for the study should be adjusted in accordance to the subjects who completed the baseline evaluation (the per protocol analysis group). A chart of patient's accountability and disposal is helpful to describe the overall accountability of the study patients, starting with patients screened and

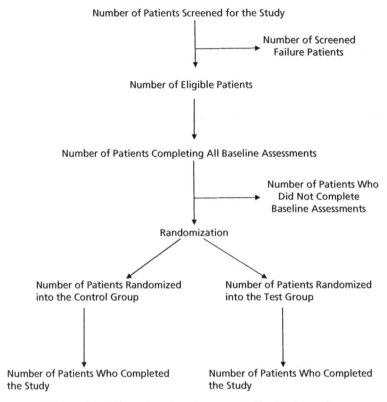

Figure 6.1   Chart of patients' accountability in the study

ending with patients who complete the study. A template for the patients accountability chart is presented in Figure 6.1.

Investigational Device Accountability

This section provides accountability for the number of devices received, used, and returned to the sponsor because of device unused, or malfunction.

Device Malfunctions/Issues/Problems

A list of all device malfunction, failures, and issues occurred in the study (description of the malfunction event, explanation of whether this event affected study data or resulted in adverse events or not, and discussion of how this malfunction event was resolved, e.g., device was removed, replaced).

When completing the primary endpoint analysis, as is going to be discussed in the subsequent section, it is important to examine if any of the subjects who met the primary endpoint had a device failure or malfunction event that resulted in the replacement of the product, or surgical intervention to retrieve the product or resolve a damage done by the product. If the patient experienced any of these events, then this patient could not be counted as a success in the study.

Analysis of the Study's Endpoints[34]

In a pivotal study the endpoints of the study are divided into primary, secondary, and sometimes other endpoints. This section starts with definition of each endpoint, and definition of success criteria. Since the study is powered on the primary endpoint(s), it is important to indicate whether the primary endpoint was met. Analyses of the primary endpoint(s) are sometimes divided into a per-protocol analysis and a per-intent-to-treat analysis. The per-protocol analysis is an analysis pertaining to patients who followed all key protocol procedures, and completed all baseline and follow-up assessments as specified in the protocol. The analysis of the primary effectiveness endpoint should be based on the per protocol analysis. The reason that the primary effective endpoint is based on the per-protocol population because the sample size of entire population should be adjusted by eliminating patients who did not follow the key protocol procedures, lost to follow-up, withdrew consent, or missing follow-up assessments, which could introduce a bias against those patients. The per-intent-to-treat-analysis is an analysis of the entire study population, including the patients who did not follow all protocol procedures, were lost to follow-up, withdrew consent, or missed follow-up evaluations. The safety analysis in the study is usually based on per-intent-to-treat analysis group.

Safety Evaluation of the Study[35]

The safety of an investigative therapy could be evaluated by determining primary safety endpoint that usually evaluates major adverse events (specific category of serious adverse events pertaining to the study and results in a residual or total damage or disability, e.g., death, stroke, myocardial infarction) and also by evaluating several other safety issues such as serious adverse events, or adverse events, or device failure/malfunctions that cause or result in an adverse event, unanticipated adverse device effects, or severe device-related adverse events. In evaluating any new therapy, it is important to know that FDA approval of the therapy depends on the evaluation of both the safety and effectiveness of this therapy.

The performed analysis detailed in this report should include a full explanation about the safety of the device such as adverse event severity: the number of AEs classified as mild, moderate, and severe in the study, the number of AEs and SAEs occurring in the study, the device- and procedure-related AEs, and any device malfunction/performance issues that results in adverse events. Any specific procedure that is used to evaluate adverse events (e.g., blind review of adverse events by clinical experts, review of major adverse events and SAE by DSMB or CEC committees) should be covered as well. A narrative of all serious and major adverse events occurring in the study would be given in this section. The narrative should include the following information, patient's age; sex; baseline prognostic risks such as diabetes, hypercholesterolemia, or heart disease; a description of the procedure performed; the success of the procedure; a description of the SAE; and the resolution and outcome of the SAE.

Subject Individual Data Sets

Listings of subject individual data sets (e.g., demographic and baseline characteristics, primary and secondary endpoint outcomes, adverse events and serious adverse events) should be provided in the final clinical report, in addition to the sum of data sets of all study subjects.

Study Compliance Analysis

As mentioned above, the success of a clinical study depends on the demonstration of the study's primary effectiveness and safety endpoints, and also on showing that compliance issues were minimal and did not raise any concern regarding data integrity, patient rights, and safety. The compliance issues analysis includes an evaluation of the following issues: consenting subject's noncompliance; protocol deviations, particularly inclusion/exclusion criteria deviations; protocol critical procedure deviations; and missing follow-up data (missing data that affected the outcome of the study).

Missing patient follow-up data can affect the outcome of the study in two ways: (1) the sample size and the pre-determined power of the study and (2) the patient population of the study if the missing data belongs to certain patient subcategory (e.g., patients who felt better or worse). The power of the study could be compromised by missing data because the sample size is used to support the primary study endpoint, missing follow-up data can have severe consequences. One way to prevent this result is to anticipate its occurrence in advance, before starting the trial, and thus to build some room in the proposed sample size for expected or potential follow-up missing data and to include 5% or 10% additional patients than what was estimated in the sample size assumptions.

To prevent extensive protocol or procedure deviations in global clinical studies, where international clinical sites are included as a part of an FDA study and final clinical report is planned to be submitted to FDA and other international regulatory authorities, it is important to coordinate the procedures in the study protocol with both US and foreign regulations whenever is possible.

Missing Data Analysis

There are different reasons for missing data in clinical studies, such as patients' withdrawal from the study, dropouts due to treatment failures or successes, and patients moving. Missing data effects on the study can range from minimal to compromising the outcome of the study such as if baseline measurements and follow-up visits are the cause. It is important to recognize that missing data can violate the strict intention-to-treat principle and impact the per protocol analysis.

Effect of Missing Data on the Study's Outcome
   - *Study Power*   A reduction in the number of valid assessments available for analysis due to incomplete data can result in the reduction of predetermined statistical power of the study.
   - *Patient Population*   Subjects who do not complete a clinical study are likely to be at the extremes: dropouts due to treatment failure or to an extremely good response. These extremes can ultimately affect the patient population of a study.
   - *Bias*   The introduction of bias into the study can relate to missing data that can alter the estimation of the treatment's effect and the comparability of the study groups.

Handling of Missing Data[36]

Analysis of Complete Cases   Ignore incomplete data and perform statistical analysis with completed data.

Imputation of Missing Data   Impute missing data that have not been recorded. To account for the bias introduced into the study, use methods of imputation that include the best—and worst-case scenarios of data analysis. Another simple way to impute missing data is to replace the unobserved measurements by values derived from other sources (e.g., other follow-up assessments).

Avoidance of Missing Data   Still the best way to dealing with missing data is to prevent it from happening in the first place. The could be done during the design of the study.

- Expand the sample size of the study to accommodate for subjects who drop out, become lost to follow-up, or withdraw consent.
- Perform sensitivity analysis of the projected missing data. This is a set of analyses showing the impacts of different methods of handling missing data on the study results.
- Compare the best and worst data analyses case scenarios.
- Compare the results of full sets of analyses.

Protocol Deviations and Violations

Protocol deviations or violations could be divided into serious and nonserious violations. Serious violations are deviations that can diminish the participants' safety, rights, welfare, or the integrity of the study and its resultant data. Protocol deviations should only be allowed in emergency cases to protect the safety of subjects of the study. Examples of potentially reportable deviations (i.e., if they place subjects at a greater risk) are informed consent improperly obtained or not obtained, subject enrolled without meeting the eligibility criteria and without prior sponsor approval, study drug or dose not administered per protocol and so increases the risk of harm to the subject, unauthorized removal of personal health records off site, or patient names showing on records submitted to the sponsor.

Deviation reports are usually forwarded to the IRB at the time of the continuing review. The deviation report sent to the IRB should include a description of the protocol deviation and corrective action plan to prevent it from re-occurring. For industry-sponsored studies the sponsor may keep a patient-specific deviation and violation log with each case report form. Sometimes protocol deviations are discovered during the monitoring visits, so the monitoring report should reflect the protocol deviations and corrective action plan to prevent these violations. A Protocol Violations Report should include the following information: a description of the protocol violation; notations of any compromise to patients' safety, or documentation that there were no safety issues; documentation of the contact with the sponsor regarding the situation and outcome; and a description of the action plan in response to the event.

Subgroup Analysis[37,38]

Study subgroups are best selected when predetermined in advance based on prognostic baseline indicators such as diabetes, hypercholesterolemia, heart failure, or high blood pressure. However, the study results of certain subgroups become only obvious after the completion of the main study and analysis of the data. Stratification of study data should be considered, particularly in nonrandomized trials to account for the subgroup baseline differences.

In addition subgroup analyses can have important implications when the effects of an investigational therapy are more profound in a particular subgroup than in the general population. For example, if the study results indicate the absence of a significant effect in the general population and the presence of a significant effect in a particular subgroup, it may be useful to design another clinical trial to show where the subgroup could benefit most from the therapy, and to utilize that subgroup as the general patient population of the second study. An example is the AMIHOT I study sponsored by TheroX Inc. The AMIHOT (Acute Myocardial Infarction with Hyperoxemic Oxygen Therapy) study was designed as a multicenter, randomized trial to evaluate the safety and effectiveness of supersaturated oxygen therapy for the treatment of AMI. In this study 269 patients with AMI for up to 24 hours were randomized either to standard therapy or standard therapy plus hyperoxemic oxygen therapy for 90 minutes. Results of study did not show overall improvement in the primary endpoint of myocardial function and recovery in overall patient population, which included a 24-hour inclusion window for both inferior and anterior AMI. However, in anterior AMI subjects treated within six hours of symptom onset, significant improvements were observed in the surrogate endpoints probably due to the early intervention to prevent AMI damage. The selection of this subgroup that benefited from this therapy is an example of a particular subgroup whose benefit brought more significance than the general population of the study. As a result this subgroup became the patient population of the subsequent clinical study, AMIHOT II trial. The AMIHOT II study was designed as a randomized, international multicenter trial to evaluate the safety and effectiveness of supersaturated oxygen therapy in the treatment of anterior AMI treated within six hours of symptom onset.

Examination of Data Across Study Sites

In device trials, center-to-center variations in a device's effect can be due to a physician's experience or training in using or implanting the device. Other explanation can include variations in the patient population, patient management, and reporting practices. A scientifically credible explanation is required to account for any variation of data across study centers. This part of the analysis also becomes important when multicenter trials are conducted, including international sites, so to any differences in data among the international sites or their quality of the health systems should be accounted for.

Multivariate Analysis[39]

This method of analysis is important in measuring the impact of more than one variable at a time while analyzing the data set, such as the impact of age, sex, baseline prognostic parameter (diabetes, hypertension, etc.) on particular outcome using regression analysis. This method of analysis is important in determinating certain risk factors in a study. Normalization of these risk factors in study groups eliminates the bias associated with these risk factors.

Study Interpretation and Conclusions

In this section the key findings of the study are summarized, and a set of recommendations are proposed to the clinical users based on these findings. Study interpretations and conclusions proceed through certain steps:

Step 1

- Focus on interpretation of study steps
- State clearly the key findings of the study
- Discuss how the study findings relate to the study hypothesis
- Show how data from the study prove or disapprove the study hypothesis
- Show if the direction and size of relationship agrees with expectations

Step 2
- Expand interpretation
- Relate results to clinical application
- Proceed from specific findings to broader inferences

Step 3
- Extend recommendations
- Relate study findings to current thinking
- Discuss other opinions
- Recommend clinical treatment based on new information obtained from the study

7

MEDICAL DEVICE REGULATIONS, COMBINATION PRODUCT, STUDY COMMITTEES, AND FDA-SPONSOR MEETINGS

Design, Execution, and Management of Medical Device Clinical Trials,
by Salah Abdel-aleem
Copyright © 2009 John Wiley & Sons, Inc.

In this chapter key FDA and ICH regulations applicable to medical devices are discussed to enable the reader to have a wide perspective of the regulations that govern medical devices. FDA regulations governing the submissions of 510K, IDE, PMA, and HDE are discussed as are the regulations regarding the emerging combination products such as drug-eluting stents and drug delivery systems. Other FDA regulations that could have significant implications on the development of clinical tasks and activities such as FDA-sponsor meetings (e.g., pre-IDE FDA meetings), special study committees (e.g., Data Safety Monitoring Board, DSMB, and Clinical Event Committee, CEC), IRB membership, function/responsibilities, HIPAA regulation rules, and bioresearch monitoring are reviewed. Because some of the medical device regulations noted are also applicable to drugs, the differences between drug and medical device clinical development are also briefly discussed in this chapter.

By nature, the subject material of the clinical trial tasks and activities is expansive. Certain topics, such as the international regulations of clinical trials, are beyond the scope of this book and are only briefly covered. Still a few references to international regulations are included, especially in the case where the sponsor of the trials is planning to include international sites as part of the US FDA study.

MEDICAL DEVICE REGULATIONS

Historic Key Device Legislation

1976 The history of device legislation goes back to 1976 when the Medical Device Amendment passed to ensure safety and effectiveness of medical devices, including diagnostic products. The amendments require manufacturers to register with FDA and follow quality control procedures. This Act required classification of devices. It led to the classification of approximately 1700 generic types of devices, grouped into 19 medical specialties: some products must have premarket approval by FDA; others must meet performance standards before marketing.

1990 Safe Medical Devices Act is passed, requiring nursing homes, hospitals, and other facilities that use medical devices to report to FDA incidents that suggest that a medical device probably caused or contributed to the death, serious illness, or serious injury of a patient.

Manufacturers are required to conduct postmarket surveillance on permanently implanted devices whose failure might cause serious harm or death, and to establish methods for tracing and locating patients depending on such devices. The act authorizes the FDA to order device product recalls and take other steps necessary to protect patient safety.

1997 The Food and Drug Administration Modernization Act (FDAMA) is passed, and the FDA is more efficient as a result, in making it easier for patients to get early access to medical products.

2002 Under the Medical Device User Fee and Modernization Act, sponsors of medical device applications now have fees assessed for evaluation, provisions are established for device establishment inspections by accredited third parties, and new requirements emerged for reprocessed single-use devices. The Office of Combination Products is formed within the Office of the Commissioner, as mandated under the Medical Device User Fee and Modernization Act, to oversee review of products that fall into multiple jurisdictions within FDA.

Types of Regulatory Documents

Regulatory documents could be classified as laws, regulations, or guidance documents.

Laws
- Passed by Congress and the President
- Statutory law
- Compliance is mandated by the Food, Drug, and Cosmetic Act

Regulations
- Established by the FDA
- Administrative law
- Code of Federal Regulations (CFR) Part 800-1299

Guidance Documents
- Written by FDA
- No legal requirement to follow guidelines

FDA Organizational Structure

The FDA consists of the following agencies:

- Center for Food, Safety, and Nutrition
- Center for Drug Evaluation and Research
- Center for Veterinary Medicine
- Center for Devices and Radiological Health
- National Center for Toxicological Research
- Center for Biologics Evaluation and Research

What the CDHR Does

The major responsibilities of the Center for Devices and Radiological Health (CDHR) are to review and approve premarket notifications [510(K)], IDE applications, HDE applications, premarket applications (PMA), and the medical device classification.

Premarket Notifications [510(K)]
- Most commonly used mechanism to bring medical devices to market
- Provides evidence that a medical device is as safe and as effective or substantially equivalent to a legally marketed device (predicate device) that was or is currently on the US market
- Application submitted ≥90 days prior to marketing

Premarket Approval—Application (PMA) and Supplements
- Used to request approval to market a Class III medical device
- May also be used to assess clinical data
- PMA submissions are reviewed by FDA on a 180-day timeline

Investigational Device Exemption (IDE)—Amendments and Supplements
- If the investigational device study presents a significant risk to the subjects, the sponsor must obtain FDA approval of an "investigational device exemption" application (IDE) under 21 CFR 812.
- The IDE must contain information on the study's investigational plan, report of prior investigations, device manufacturing details, IRB actions, investigator agreements, subject informed consent form, device labeling, cost of the device, and other matters related to the study.
- The IDE applies to all clinical device investigations to determine safety and effectiveness.

IDE Amendments
- All submissions related to an original IDE that have been submitted, but not approved, are referred to as "IDE amendments."
- Identification of IDE amendments enables FDA to track each IDE from the time it is originally submitted until the time it is approved.

IDE Supplements
- The sponsor of an investigation of a device with significant risk may submit a supplemental application it, for example, there is a change in the investigational plan when such a change can affect the scientific soundness of the study or the rights, safety, or welfare of the subjects
- Addition of investigational sites includes post-approval reports on unanticipated adverse effects of the device; recall and device disposition; failure to obtain informed consent; and annual progress reports, final reports, investigator lists, and other reports requested by FDA

Humanitarian Device Exemption (HDE)   A humanitarian use device (HUD) is intended to treat or diagnose diseases that affect fewer than 4000 individuals a year in the United States. HUD determination is made by FDA's Office of Orphan Products Development. HUDs can be marketed after FDA approval of a Humanitarian Device Exemption (HDE) that demonstrates device safety and probable benefit.

IRB Involvement with HDEs
- HUDs can only be used at institutions where IRBs can oversee the use of the device
- IRB must initially approve use of HUD
  - After HDE approval
  - After policy for HUD use is established
- IRB should conduct continuing review of HUD use
- Expediting the review may be an appropriate action

Classification of Medical Devices   Medical devices can be classified (regulatory classification) into the following categories.

Class I Devices (General Controls)   Examples are elastic bandages, examination gloves, and hand-held surgical instruments.

- Subject to the least amount of regulatory control
- Requiring 510(K) application if they are not exempt
- Often simpler in design than Class II or III

Class II (General Controls and Special Controls)   Examples are powered wheelchairs, infusion pumps, and surgical drapes.

- Requiring more regulatory control than Class I
- Have special labeling requirements, mandatory performance standards, and postmarket surveillance

Class III (Premarket Approval)   This most stringent regulatory category requires sufficient evidence to ensure safety and effectiveness. Examples are replacement heart valves, silicone gel-filled breast implants, and implanted cerebella stimulators.

- Supports or sustains human life
- Is substantially involved in preventing impairment of human health
- Presents a potential or unreasonable risk of illness or injury

Summary of 510(K) Process

The 510(K) premarket notification submission allows the manufacturer to demonstrate that a device is substantially equivalent to a currently marketed predicate device at least in one of these parameters:

- Materials
- Design
- Technology
- Intended use
- Performance device

Regulatory Pathways to Market: 510(K) and PMA Compared

510(K) Premarket Notification Substantial Equivalence
- Safety and effectiveness to a predicate device
- Intended use and design approval

510(K) Premarket Notification—Practical Points
- 90-day review cycle by FDA
- Data from clinical studies included if clinically required

Premarket Approval Application (PMA)   Approval is based on:
- Valid scientific evidence
- Safe (benefit outweighs risk)
- Effective (clinically significant result)

Premarket Approval Application—Practical Points
- 180-day review cycle
- Data from clinical studies usually included
- Input from independent advisory panel
- Pre-approval inspection of manufacturing facility
- Careful labeling review
- Post-approval studies

510(K) Requirements: Risk/Benefit

Risk/Benefit Ratio   The risk refers to the measure of device's *safety*; the benefit refers to the measure of the device's *acute efficacy* and *durability*.

- Substantial equivalence based on risk/benefit that does not require *equal* risks and *equal* benefits
- Device can be safer but less effective than predicate device
- Device can be less safe but more effective than predicate device

510 (K) "Substantial Equivalence" Decision-Making Process   21 CFR 807 Subpart E describes the requirements for a 510(K) submission. The process of 510(K)'s "substantial equivalence" decision-making process is presented in the flowchart shown in Figure 7.1.

As the flowchart shows, the 510(K) "substantial equivalence" decision-making process compares submissions of new devices with marketed devices. FDA requires additional information if the relationship between the marketed and "predicate" (pre-amendments or reclassified postamendments) devices is unclear. The decision tree poses questions, and the yes or no response determines the path through the flowchart. Step 1: Does the new device have the same indication statement? If the response is yes, go to Step 3. If no, follow Step 2. Step 2: Do the differences alter the intended therapeutic/diagnostic, etc., effect (in deciding, you may consider impact on safety and effectiveness)? (This decision is normally based on descriptive information alone, but limited testing information is sometimes required.) If the response is yes, the new device has a new intended use, and the device is

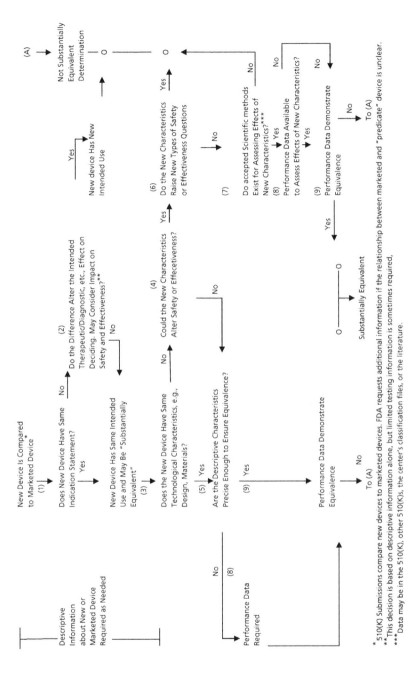

Figure 7.1 510(K) "substantial equivalence" decision-making process

New Device Is Compared to Marketed Device*
(1)

Does New Device Have Same Indication Statement?

Yes

New Device Has Same Intended Use and May Be "Substantially Equivalent"
(3)

No

Do the Difference Alter the Intended Therapeutic/Diagnostic, etc., Effect on Deciding. May Consider Impact on Safety and Effectiveness?**
(2)

Yes

New device Has New Intended Use

No

Does the New Device Have Same Technological Characteristics, e.g., Design, Materials?

Yes

No

Could the New Characteristics Alter Safety or Effectiveness?
(4)

Yes

Do the New Characteristics Raise New Types of Safety or Effectiveness Questions
(6)

Yes

No

Are the Descriptive Characteristics Precise Enough to Ensure Equivalence?
(5)

Yes

No

Do accepted Scientific methods Exist for Assessing Effects of New Characteristics?***
(7)

No

Yes

Performance Data Available to Assess Effects of New Characteristics?
(8)

Yes

No

Descriptive Information about New or Marketed Device Required as Needed

Performance Data Required
(8)

No

Performance Data Demonstrate Equivalence
(9)

Yes

Performance Data Demonstrate Equivalence
(9)

No

To (A)

Yes

Substantially Equivalent

Not Substantially Equivalent Determination
(A)

No

To (A)

* 510(K) Submissions compare new devices to marketed devices. FDA requests additional information if the relationship between marketed and "predicate" device is unclear.
** This decision is based on descriptive information alone, but limited testing information is sometimes required,
*** Data may be in the 510(K)s, other 510(K)s, the center's classification files, or the literature.

135

determined not substantially equivalent. If the response is no, proceed to Step 3. The new device has the same intended use and may be "substantially equivalent." Step 3: Does the new device have the same technological characteristics, e.g., design, materials? If the response is yes, proceed to Step 5.

If the response is no, proceed to Step 4. Step 4: Could the new characteristics affect safety or effectiveness? If the response is no, proceed to Step 5. If yes, proceeded to Step 6. Step 6: Do the new characteristics raise new types of safety or effectiveness questions. If the response is yes, the device is determined not substantially equivalent. If the response is no, proceed to Step 7. Step 7: Do accepted scientific methods exist for assessing effects of the new characteristics? If the response is no, the device is determined not substantially equivalent. If yes, proceed to Step 8. Step 8: Are performance data available to assess effects of new characteristics? (Data may be in the 510(K), other 510(K)s, the Center's classification files, or the literature.) Proceed to Step 9. Step 9: Does the performance data demonstrate equivalence? If the response is no, the device is determined not substantially equivalent. If yes, the device is determined "substantially equivalent."

Back to Step 5: Are the descriptive characteristics precise enough to ensure equivalence? If the response is yes, the device is determined substantially equivalent. If no, proceed to Step 8. Step 8: Are the performance data available to assess equivalence? If the response is no, performance data is required. Proceed to Step 9. Step 9: Does the performance data demonstrate equivalence? If the response is no, the device is determined not substantially equivalent. If the response is yes, the device is determined to be substantially equivalent.

510(K) Postmarket Issues   FDA can require postmarket surveillance of 510(K) cleared devices (21 CFR Section 522)
Device must be:

- Likely to have serious adverse health consequences as a result of failure
- Intended for at least one year of implantation
- Life-sustaining

Product Codes

Product codes are classifications for individual device types. These codes are found in 21 CFR parts 862–892. If there is more than one class in a regulation, then there is more than one product code. Product codes are on FDA letters and are available on the internet.

- Used to describe device types existing prior to May 28, 1976
- Classified by premarket review
- New uses or new technologies assigned new product codes (most product codes are put under a classification regulation)
- Found on all 510(K)/PMA clearance/approval letters
- Ultimately classify the device
- Used to search for a predicate device
- Used in assigning inspections
- Used to search medical device reports (MDRs) in public database
- Used to search listings in public database

The CDRH only releases product codes for cleared/approved device types or for devices intended only export use.

GMDN Codes   The Global Medical Device Nomenclature (GMDN) is a collection of terms each with a unique code number to describe and catalog medical devices (Table 7.1). GMDN was developed in accordance to the International Standards Organization (EN ISO 15225).

GMDN is a three-tiered system consisting of 12 categories of devices grouped as follows:

- Template terms. By generic device groups identified with its unique code
- Preferred terms. By product type (e.g., model type).

The 12 GMDN Device Categories

TABLE 7.1   Categories in the GMDN Code Table

Code	Term
01	Active implantable devices
02	Anesthetic and respiratory devices
03	Dental devices
04	Electromechanical devices
05	Hospital hardware
06	In vitro diagnostic devices
07	Non-active implantable devices
08	Ophthalmic and optical devices
09	Reusable instruments
10	Single use devices
11	Technical aids for disabled persons
12	Diagnostic and therapeutic radiation devices

CDRH Advisory Committees
- Medical Device Advisory Committee (18 panels)
- Device Good Manufacturing Practice (GMP) Advisory Committee
- National mammography Quality Assurance Advisory Committee
- Technical Electronic Product Radiation Safety Standard Committee

FDA Advisory Panels

The FDA assembled 18 advisory panels:

1. Anesthesiology and Respiratory Therapy Devices
2. Circulatory System Devices
3. Clinical Chemistry and Clinical Toxicology Devices
4. Dental Products
5. Ear, Nose, and Throat Devices
6. Gastroenterology and Urology Devices
7. General and Plastic Surgery Devices
8. General Hospital and Personal Use Devices
9. Hematology and Pathology Devices
10. Immunology Devices
11. Medical Device Dispute Resolution
12. Microbiology Devices
13. Molecular and Clinical Genetic
14. Neurological Devices
15. Obstetrics and Gynecology Devices
16. Ophthalmic Devices
17. Orthopedic and Rehabilitation devices
18. Radiological Devices

Roles and Functions of FDA Advisory Panels
- Each panel is made up of experts in the field including physicians, surgeons, scientists, engineers, consumer representatives, and industry representatives (nonvoting members).
- The panels review relevant submissions to FDA and make recommendations to the FDA to accept or reject, based on a vote.
- At the panel meeting the sponsor makes a presentation to the panel to support the submission.

- The FDA may choose to accept or reject the panel recommendation.
- One of the initial roles of the FDA panel was to determine the classification of devices into Class I, II, or III.

The panel also makes recommendations regarding whether a device should have its class designation downgraded.

Summary of PMA Process

Premarket approval (PMA) applications must demonstrate a reasonable assurance of safety and effectiveness for a device based on its intended use.

- PMA process reserved for Class III devices (highest risk, e.g., pacemakers)
- Clinical data provided in most PMA submissions
- Review time by the FDA is typically 180 days

PMA Postmarket Issues FDA can require postmarket studies for PMA-approved devices. This requisition is normally put in the PMA approval notification among other conditions of PMA approval. The postmarket studies proposed by the FDA consider risks and benefits of premarket and postmarket data collection on the device's availability compared with clinical evidence during its development.

The post-approval study conditions agreed upon by the PMA sponsor and the FDA may include:

- Collection of data from new patients
- Collection of data from existing patients
- Enhanced analysis of adverse event data
- IRB review and approval of post-FDA approved study clinical protocols

PMA Submission The PMA can be submitted as one of the following:

Modular
- Preclinical data
- Manufacturing details
- Clinical details

Traditional
  • Expanded IDE
  • Full description of clinical results

Streamlined PMA, Product Development Protocol, or Humanitarian Device Exemption (HDE)
  • Device intended use for <4000 US pts/year
  • Only need to show safety data

What Happens after PMA Submission?   The FDA response time to PMA submission can be summarized as follows:

  • Filing decision—within 45 days
  • Review cycle—technically 180 days
    • In-depth review
    • Panel meeting possible
  • Audits
    • Bioresearch monitoring (BIMO)
      • Clinical site and IRB
      • Preclinical site
    • Quality system inspection

Device Risk Classification

To be classified as a significant risk (SR) device, one of the following features must be present:

  • A potential by serious risk to subject health, safety, or welfare
  • Intended as an implant
  • Used in supporting or sustaining human life
  • Substantial importance in diagnosing, curing, mitigating, or treating disease, or otherwise prevents impairment of human health

All other devices are classified as having *nonsignificant risk* (NSR)

Determination Nonsignificant Risk Medical Devices   The assessment of whether a device presents a nonsignificant risk (NSR) is initially made by the sponsor. The IRB may agree or disagree with the sponsor's initial NSR assessment. The IRB serves, in a sense, as the FDA's surrogate with respect to review and approval of NSR studies.

If a reviewing IRB agrees with the sponsor's designation of a device study as NSR, the investigation may begin at that institution immediately, without an IDE application to the FDA.

NSR device studies, however, should not be confused with the concept of "minimal risk," a term utilized in the Institutional Review Board (IRB) regulations (21 CFR Part 56) to identify certain studies that may be approved through an "expedited review" procedure. For both SR and NSR device studies, IRB approval prior to conducting clinical trials and continuing the review by the IRB are required. In addition informed consent must be obtained for either type of study (21 CFR Part 50).

Nonsignificant Risk Studies   Nonsignificant risk studies must follow abbreviated IDE regulations (21 CFR 812.2(b)):

- IRB approval
- Labeling
- Informed consent
- Monitoring and records
- Prohibition against promotion

Minimal Risk   It should be noted that the term "minimal risk" is not equivalent to nonsignificant risk. Minimal risk studies are nonsignificant risk studies that present *no more than minimal risk* to subjects. This may include harm and discomfort not greater than ordinarily encountered in one's everyday life or in routine medical exams. Minimal risk studies are subject to expedited IRB review (21 CFR 56.110).

CMS (Centers for Medicare and Medicaid Services) Categorization
- FDA provides CMS relevant information about the investigational devices included in each IDE it approves
- FDA aids CMS in making "reasonable and necessary" coverage determinations for investigational devices

Experimental Devices   Device can be classified as experimental or nonexperimental. *It should be noted that the term experimental device is not equivalent to investigational device.*

Experimental devices have unanswered initial safety and effectiveness questions:

- Completely new device type
- "Absolute risk" not yet established

Category A—Experimental
- A1: Class III device for which no PMA has been approved for any indicated use
- A2: Class III device that would be Category B (nonexperimental) but has undergone significant modifications for a new intended use

Category B—nonexperimental
- B1: Device under investigation to determine substantial equivalence (510(K) expected)
- B2: Class III device with similar technology and intended use to currently marketed device
- B3: Class III device with technological advances compared to marketed device (next generation)
- B4: Class III device comparable to marketed device under investigation for a new intended use
- B5: Pre-amendment Class III device for which no PMA has been approved
- B6: Nonsignificant risk device for which FDA requires an IDE

Categorization Information
- CMS does not reimburse for experimental devices
- Categorization determination is confidential
- Sponsor may request reconsideration
- FDA may change categorization if new information becomes available
- Example of a reimbursable device: PMA for comparable device approved

IDE Approval versus Disapproval

An IDE application that is submitted to the FDA could be approved, approved with conditions, or disapproved by the FDA:

IDE Approval   The FDA has no concerns about device safety or the validity of the clinical data to be collected.

IDE Conditional Approval   The FDA may conditionally approve an IDE if there are outstanding questions regarding the device or the proposed study that do not involve device safety. In the case of IDE conditional approval, the sponsor must respond to the FDA's concerns within 45 days.

IDE Disapproval   The FDA has significant concerns about device safety or the scientific soundness of the proposed study that prevent initiation of the clinical study.

Similarities and Differences Between Medical Devices and Pharmaceutical Clinical Trials

The clinical development process of drugs and medical devices has several similarities and differences because of the nature and mechanism of action of the product. A common regulatory goal is that the market approval of the product is based on providing evidence for safety and efficacy of these products.

Difference between drugs and medical devices exist in the following areas:

- Nature of the Product
- Product Classification
- Mechanism of Action
- Product Development
- Length of Time & Funds
- Pre-clinical Differences
- Different Regulatory Pathways for Product Approval
- Clinical Trial Design Differences
- Post-approval Differences

Nature of the Product-Definitions of Drugs & Devices

Drugs
- Articles other than food listed in the U.S. Pharmacopoeia, U.S. Homoeopathic Pharmacopoeia, or National Formulary
- Intended to diagnose, cure, mitigate, treat, or prevent disease
- Affect the structure & function of the human body

Devices
- An instrument, apparatus, implement, machine, implant, or in vitro reagent listed in the U,S. Pharmacopoeia or National Formulary
- Does not achieve primary effect through chemical action
- Is not dependent on being metabolized
- Includes device/drug and device/biologic combinations
- Three classes of devices based on risk and required controls

Device Classification
- **Class I (General Controls)**
  - Low risk devices—general controls only (reasonable assurance of the safety and effectiveness
  - Require 510k application if they are not exempt
  - Are often simpler in design than Class II or III
  - Examples: Elastic bandages, examination gloves, and hand-held surgical instruments
- **Class II (General Controls & Special Controls)**
  - Require more regulatory control than Class I
  - Special labeling requirements, mandatory performance standards and post-market surveillance
  - Examples: powered wheelchairs, infusion pumps, and surgical drapes
- **Class III (Premarket Approval)**
  - Most stringent regulatory category that requires sufficient evidence to assure safety and effectiveness
  - Supports or sustains human life, is substantially involved in preventing impairment of human health, or presents a potential or unreasonable risk of illness or injury
  - Clinical data & pre-market approval required
  - Examples: replacement heart valves, silicone gel-filled breast implants and implanted cerebella stimulators

Mechanism of Action
- Devices and drugs have different mechanisms of action:
  - Local device versus drug systemic effects
  - Physical effects for devices versus pharmacokinetic effects of drugs

Length of Time & Funds   Generally speaking the process of drug development requires more time and funds than that of medical devices. The drug development process requires Pre-clinical, clinical development (Phase I, II, and III), FDA approval, and post-market approval phase. This process may take an average of 20 years. On the other hand, the device development process requires design of the product, pre-clinical testing, human clinical trials (Feasibility and pivotal studies), FDA approval, and may also require post-market evaluation. This Process takes an average of 8–10 years.

Drug & Device Regulation   Drugs and devices are both regulated by the US Food and Drug Administration. The FDA regulation of drugs started earlier than devices (1938 for drugs versus 1976 for devices). Drugs are regulated by the Center for Drug Evaluation and Research (CDER) and regulated by 21 CFR part *312* (investigational drugs) and 21 CFR part *314* (market approval). On the other hand, devices are regulated by Center for Devices and Radiological Health (CDRH) and regulated by 21 CFR part *812* (investigational devices) and 21 CFR part *814* (market approval). However, the following regulations are common to both drugs and devices: 21 CFR part 50 (Protection of Human Subjects), 21 CFR part 56 (Institutional Review Boards), 21 CFR part 54 (Financial Disclosure), 21 CFR part 11 (Electronic Records), and HIPAA Privacy Rule.

Investigational Product Applications

Drugs (part 312)

- Investigational New Drug (IND)
- IND must be submitted prior to conducting a clinical investigation with an investigational drug (312.20)
- Exemptions (312.2b)

Devices (part 812)

- Investigational Device Exemption (IDE)
- IDE required prior to conducting a clinical investigation (812.20)
- *Two paths*: significant vs non-significant risk studies
- Exemptions (812.2c)
- Both are requests for exemption from Federal law prohibiting shipment of an unapproved drug or device in interstate commerce
- Both also permit use of product in a clinical study to collect safety and efficacy data

IND Exemptions and IDE exemptions may include the following parameters:

IND Exemptions

- Lawfully marketed in the US
- Not intended to support a new indication
- Not intended to support a change in advertising
- Doesn't involve a factor that increases risk of use

- Conducted in compliance with IRB (part 56) and Informed Consent (part 50) requirements
- Complies with the requirements for promotion and charging of investigational drugs (312.7)

IDE Exemptions

- Use in accordance with indications
- Non-invasive diagnostic
- Consumer preference testing
- Solely for veterinary use
- Research on or with lab animals
- Custom device (not being used to determine safety and efficacy for commercial distribution)

IDE Decision Process

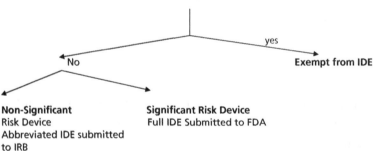

Approved for commercial release & used according to labeling or otherwise exempt

yes

No

Exempt from IDE

Non-Significant
Risk Device
Abbreviated IDE submitted
to IRB

Significant Risk Device
Full IDE Submitted to FDA

IND Content   The IND application contains the following contents:

- Form FDA 1571
- Investigational plan
- Investigator brochure
- Clinical Protocols (study, investigator, facilities, IRB)
- Chemistry, manufacturing, control data
- Environmental impact statement
- Pharmacology and toxicology data
- Previous human experience
- Report of prior investigations

- Case report forms
- Risk analysis
- Description of the product
- Monitoring procedures
- Manufacturing information & environmental impact
- Investigator information
- Sales information
- Labeling
- Informed consent materials and IRB information

IDE Content   See Section Under "IDE Deliverables" in this chapter.

Marketing Applications   The following marketing applications exist for drugs and medical devices;

Drugs (part 314)

- New Drug Application (NDA)
- Supplemental NDA
- Abbreviated NDA—generics

Devices (part 814)

- Premarket approval application (PMA)—Class III devices
- Supplemental PMA
- 510(K)—Class II devices

Clinical Study Design Differences   A fundamental difference between drugs and devices clinical study differences is that a single confirmatory trial for devices. Whereas, The standard for the approval of a pharmaceutical drug regulation is based on two well-controlled Phase III trials that demonstrate the safety and efficacy of the drug. Other differences between the clinical study design of drugs and devices may include the following:

- Feasibility & pivotal studies for devices versus Phase I–III for drugs
- Fewer subjects for device trials due to large effect size: a typical pivotal device study includes 500–1000 subjects versus 1000–3000 subjects in pivotal drug study.

- Shorter participation in device trials (but may be subject to post-market study): the duration of subject follow up in devices is shorter than that of drugs. However, some medical post-approval studies are required to evaluate long-term effects of the devices (it could take up to 5 years in some post-market studies).
- Placebo control versus "sham" control
- Device trials may not be randomized or may employ device features: the golden standard design is a randomized study for both drugs and devices, but sometimes is difficult to adopt this design because of ethical concern
- Blinding/masking often not possible with devices
- Device technology may change during the study

A great deal of similarities exist between drugs and medical devices regarding the sponsor responsibilities, selection of investigators, selection of study monitors, monitoring investigations, reporting of adverse events, investigator responsibilities, and record retention.

Sponsor Responsibilities

Drugs (312.50–52)

- Select qualified investigators
- Ensure proper monitoring
- Can transfer obligations to a CRO

Devices (812.40)

- *Same as drug but* No language on "transfer of obligations" to CRO

Selecting Investigators

Drugs (312.53)

- Select investigators qualified by training and experience
- Ship investigational product (IP) only to participating investigators
- Obtain investigator information (CV, Form FDA 1572, financial)

Devices (812.43)

- *Same as drug but* No 1572: but similar information are listed in Investigator agreement instead

Selecting Monitors

Drugs (312.53d)

- Select monitors qualified by training and experience to monitor the investigation

Devices (812.43d)

- *Same as drug*

Monitoring Investigations

Drugs (312.56)

- If non-compliance discovered, secure compliance or discontinue IP shipments, terminate participation, and dispose/return of IP
- Disqualification by FDA (312.70)
- Discontinue investigations if IP presents an unreasonable risk

Devices (812.46)

- *Same as drug but*
- Don't dispose/return device if it would jeopardize subject (eg., explant)
- Disqualification by FDA (812.119)
- Can resume terminated studies of significant risk device only after FDA and IRB approval

Sponsor Reporting to FDA

Drugs

- Protocol amendments (312.30) and IND amendments (312.31)
- IND Safety Reports of serious & unexpected drug-related adverse events (312.32)
- IND Annual Reports (312.33)
- New investigators reported as part of protocol amendments

Devices

- IDE supplemental applications (812.35)
- IDE Safety Reports of serious & Unanticipated adverse device effects—UADE (812.150b)

- Annual progress reports and final report, if significant risk device (812.150b)
- Current investigator list every 6-months
- Significant risk determination by IRB
- Any sponsor request for device return, repair, or disposition (e.g., recall)
- Withdrawal IRB approval

Unanticipated Adverse Device Effect (21 CFR 812.3r)   Serious adverse effect on health or safety or any life-threatening problem or death caused by, or associated with a device, if that effect, problem, or death was not previously identified in nature, severity, or degree of incidence in the investigational plan or application, or any other unanticipated serious problem associated with a device that relates to the rights, safety or welfare of patients.

Sponsor Record Retention

Drugs (312.57)

- Maintain investigator records including financial disclosure
- Maintain records of IP shipment/disposition
- Retention for 2 years after market approval or investigational use is discontinued

Devices (812.140)

- *Same as drug but*
- Retention for 2 years after no longer needed to support a market approval application

Investigator Responsibilities

Drugs (312.360)

- Ensure investigation conducted according to investigational plan and FDA regulations
- Protect rights, safety, welfare of subjects
- Ensure informed consent obtained per part 50

Devices (812.100)

- *Same as drug plus*

• Language permitting *potential subject recruitment* (e.g., interest), but not consent, prior to IRB and FDA approval (812.110)

Special Device and Drug Challenges Issues
1. Obtaining Informed Consent
   a. Timing of informed consent can be difficult as subjects often enroll on same day of treatment (non-elective patient enrollment)
   b. Indications for use of specific device may not be confirmed until sometime during a surgical procedure
   c. Subjects may require pre-medication for treatment
   d. Investigator skill and training with equipment varies
   e. Investigator training on device use may be difficult due to influx of new residents and fellows and rapid changes in technology
2. Device Accountability
   a. Monitoring and controlling device inventory may be difficult due to storage location (i.e., O.R. supply room) and device size/portability.
   b. Some devices require "multi-use" accountability
   c. Changes in device technology during trial may require frequent inventory changes
3. Drug/Device Administration
   a. Drugs (312.61)
      i. Administer IP to subjects under personal supervision or supervision of sub-investigator
      ii. Supply IP only to authorized persons
   b. Devices (812.110c)
      i. *Same as drug but*
      ii. Permit device to be used with subjects under investigator's supervision—no language about delegation to others
4. Records Inspection by FDA
   a. Drugs (312.58, 68)
      i. Sponsors and investigators will permit FDA to access, copy, and verify all records related to clinical investigations
      ii. Investigator records may identify subjects if FDA finds necessary
   b. Devices (812.145)
      i. *Same as drug*

TABLE 7.2 Device Approvals in Different Regions in the World

Country/Region	Premarket	Placing on Market
United States	PMA or 510(K) marketing clearance	Establishment registration
European Union	Compliance label CE mark	Responsible person registration
Japan[a]	*Shonin* (approval) or *todokede* (notification)	Seizo-gyo (manufacturer license) *Yunyu hanbai-gyo* (Import License) *Hanbai todoke* (sales notification)
Canada	Device license	Establishment license
Australia[b]	ARTG number	Enterprise identification (ENTID)

[a]Japan's PAL (Pharmaceutical Administration Law).
[b]Australia's new medical devices legislation was passed by the Australian Parliament in April 2002.

Device Approval in Different World Regions   Authorities acknowledge product clearance for the market in various ways (Table 7.2).

In Europe, all products entering European Union (EU) markets should bear the self-declared CE marking to demonstrate compliance with relevant EU directives. For medical devices, applicable EU Directives include the Active Implantable Medical Devices Directive (AIMDD, 90/385/EEC), the Medical Devices Directive (MDD, 93/42/EEC), and the In-vitro Diagnostic Devices Directive (IVDD, 98/79/EC).

In Australia, the Therapeutic Goods Administration issues an ARTG (Australian Register of Therapeutic Goods) number to devices cleared for the market.

In Canada, a Device License is awarded by the Therapeutic Products Directorate. In the European Union, after receiving the EC certificate from a notified body, the manufacturer places the CE mark on or with the device.

In Japan, the healthcare system is dramatically different from that of the United States. The Japanese government imposes stringent regulatory procedures for certifications of new medical devices from foreign countries. To obtain device approval in Japan, the manufacturer must first obtain two documents from the Ministry of Health, Labor and Welfare (MHLW)—the *kyoka* (license) and the *shonin* (premarket approval). A foreign manufacturer must appoint a representative who has a license to sell medical devices in Japan. Both the foreign and domestic representatives are responsible for all applicable regulatory compliance with regard to imported procedures and documents, GMPs and postmarketing surveillance. There are three risk classes (from low to high risk) in Japan.

Device Trial Management Issues   The following are topics or issues that need to be addressed prior to or during the course of clinical trials:

- Study contracts
- Medicare national coverage decision
- Unanticipated adverse device effects (UADE) versus serious adverse events/adverse events (SAE/AE)
- Who pays for the device?
- Investigator training/proctoring

Study Contracts   The following are examples of certain long-term follow-up procedures that are not considered standard practice but the cost of which should still be considered by the clinical site when signing the contract with the study sponsor:

- Patient follow-up could require extended long-term and postmarket surveillance for up to 5 years.
- Patients may be required to have more invasive testing to ensure device efficacy, such as repeat angiography/IVUS for DES.

For a more detailed discussion on study contracts, see Chapter 1.

Who Pays for the Device?   Medicare will provide reimbursement for covered individuals in the setting of a device clinical trial, if *the device is categorized as a type B in the IDE.*

Although medicare may reimburse for the device, local private payers may not. So prior authorization is needed.

Unanticipated Adverse Device Effects (UADE) versus Serious Adverse Events/Adverse Events (SAE/AE)   Sometimes it is challenging to decide whether an adverse event in a particular study is a serious adverse event or a serious unanticipated adverse device effect. Development of a list of potential AEs in the clinical protocol could therefore be helpful in resolving the issue. If there is a disagreement as to whether an SAE is anticipated or unanticipated, the DSMB or the Clinical Event Adjudication committee should be consulted. For more detail on this subject, see Chapter 4.

IDE Deliverables   The IDE contains several tasks pertaining to pre-clinical development, manufacturing, clinical investigations, and so forth. The key deliverables in the IDE are listed below:

Investigator Brochure
- Clinical study design
- Device description
- Report of prior investigations
  - Prior clinical research
  - Animal studies
  - Bench testing and qualification testing
- Hazard analysis
- Manufacturing and quality control
- Labeling

Investigational Plan
- Purpose
- Device description
- Protocol
- Risk/benefit analysis
- Monitoring procedures
- Adverse events
- Draft labeling
- Draft informed consent form
- IRB information
- Other Participating Institutions

Case Report Forms

Clinical Investigators
- List of investigators
- Investigator CVs
- Financial disclosure
- Investigator agreement letter

Appendixes
- IFU
- Bibliography/articles

Discussion of Some Clinical Deliverables in the IDE

Report of Prior Investigations   A report of prior investigations must include reports of all prior published and unpublished clinical, animal, and laboratory testing of the device. It should be comprehensive and sufficient to justify the proposed investigation.

Specificably contents of the report should include the following items:

- A bibliography of all publications that are relevant to an evaluation of the safety and effectiveness of the device
- Copies of all published and unpublished adverse information
- Copies of other significant publications if requested by an IRB or FDA
- A summary of all other unpublished information (whether adverse or supportive) that is relevant to an evaluation of the safety and effectiveness of the device
- If nonclinical laboratory data are provided, a statement that such studies has been conducted in compliance with the good laboratory practice (GLP) regulation in 21 CFR Part 58. If the study was not conducted in compliance with the GLP regulation, include a brief statement of the reason for noncompliance.

Investigational Plan   The investigational plan must include the following items in the following order:

- Purpose. This section briefly defines the patient population, intended use, and the objectives and duration of the investigation.
- Device Description. A detailed description of the device should include its various components and accessories including pictures and diagrams.
- Protocol. In the written protocol the details of the selection of the patient population are described as determined by specific inclusion/exclusion criteria, methodology to be used in the study (baseline, procedure, and follow-up assessments), study objectives, and endpoints.
- Risk Analysis. A description and analysis are provided of all higher than minimal risks to the research subjects and how these risks will be minimized.

- Monitoring procedures. The sponsor's written procedures for monitoring the investigation and the name and address of each monitor are given.
- A description of the methods, facilities, and controls used for the manufacture, processing, packing, storage, and installation of the device.
- An example of the agreement to be signed by the investigators and a list of the names and addresses of all investigators. Information that must be included in the written agreement is as follows:
  - Certification that all investigators have signed the agreement, that the list of investigators includes all investigators participating in the study, and that new investigators will sign the agreement before being added to the study
  - A list of the names, addresses, and chairpersons of all IRBs that have or will be asked to review the investigation and a certification of IRB action concerning the investigation (when available)
  - The name and address of any institution (other than those above) where a part of the investigation may be conducted (e.g., a Core lab)
  - The amount, if any, charged for the device and an explanation of why the sale does not constitute commercialization
- Copies of all labeling for the device
- Copies of all informed consent forms and all related information materials to be provided to subjects as required by 21 CFR 50, Protection of Human Subjects.

Any other relevant information that FDA requests for review of the IDE application.

Reimbursement

Reimbursement for newly approved devices could be established through:

- Already existing devices that have pathways for reimbursement already established
- New devices (and some improved devices) that need to establish reimbursement. These devices must have established:
  - Codes (CPT, ICD9, etc.)
  - Coverage

- Possible insurers
  - Government: Medicare (CMS)
  - Private insurers

Principles of ICH GCP

The principles of ICH good clinical practice (GCP) regarding the conduct of clinical trials could be summarized in the following points:

1. Clinical trials should be conducted in accordance with the ethical principles described in the Declaration of Helsinki, and that are consistent with GCP and the applicable regulatory requirement(s).

2. Before a trial is initiated, foreseeable risks and inconveniences should be weighed against the anticipated benefit for the individual trial subject and/or society. A trial should be initiated and continued only if the anticipated benefits justify the risks.

3. The rights, safety, and well-being of the trial subjects are the most important considerations and should prevail over interests of science and society.

4. The available nonclinical and clinical information on an investigational product should be adequate to support the proposed clinical trial.

5. Clinical trials should be scientifically sound, and described in a clear, detailed protocol.

6. A trial should be conducted in compliance with the protocol that has received prior institutional review board (IRB)/independent ethics committee (IEC) approval/favorable opinion.

7. The medical care given to, and medical decisions made on behalf of, subjects should always be the responsibility of a qualified physician.

8. Each individual involved in conducting a trial should be qualified by education, training, and experience to perform his or her respective task(s).

9. Freely given informed consent should be obtained from every subject prior to clinical trial participation.

10. All clinical trial information should be recorded, handled, and stored in a way that allows its accurate reporting, interpretation, and verification.

11. The confidentiality of records that could identify subjects should be protected, respecting the privacy and confidentiality rules in accordance with the applicable regulatory requirement(s).
12. Investigational products should be manufactured, handled, and stored in accordance with applicable good manufacturing practice (GMP). They should be used in accordance with the approved protocol.
13. Systems with procedures that ensure the quality of every aspect of the trial should be implemented.

Regulation of Medical Devices and Drugs Compared

The standard for the approval of a pharmaceutical drug regulation is based on two well-controlled Phase III trials that demonstrate the safety and efficacy of the drug. The standard for medical devices also depends on a regulatory pathway, but is usually is based on not more than one confirmatory, well-controlled multicenter study.

There are several differences between device and drug clinical trials. Key differences are associated with the plan and conduct of the pivotal study. The device pivotal study has a sample size ranging from 500 to 1000 subjects, while a drug pivotal study is comprised of two studies ranging 1000 to 3000 subjects.

The clinical trial phases for an investigational drug can be summarized as follows:

Phase I Studies (Clinical Pharmacology and Toxicology)
- Small sample size studies (20–80 subjects) and usually conduced in healthy volunteers
- No control group
- Usually open label
- Mainly conducted to evaluate safety and not efficacy of the drug
- Mainly to determine an acceptable single dose without causing any serious side effects
- Information obtained from dose-escalation experiments, whereby volunteers receive increasing doses of the drug according to a predetermined schedule

Phase II Studies (Initial Clinical Investigation for the Treatment Effect)
- Fairly small-scale studies.
- Aimed at the safety and efficacy of the drug with the following specific goals:

- "Proof of principal phase"
- Accurate identification of patient population that can benefit from the drug
- Verification of dosing regimen's efficacy determined in Phase I studies

Phase III Studies (Full-scale Evaluation of Treatment)
- Large trial involving substantial number of patients
- Comparison of experimental drug with current standard therapy
- Multiple centers involved
- Double-blind studies used whenever is possible

Phase IV Studies (Postmarket Surveillance)
- Very large scale clinical trials
- Occur after the approval of the drug
- Monitor adverse events and capture rare adverse events

Class III Medical Devices Class III medical devices are usually evaluated in three phases of trials:

Phase I: Feasibility, Pilot Study
- Confirm design and operating specifications
- Establish parameters for pivotal study (e.g., sample size, success criteria)
- Must have valid scientific objective
- Small sample size (10–50 patients)

Phase II: Pivotal Trial
- Demonstrate safety and effectiveness of device
- Confirm Indication for use
- Typically multicenter, randomized controlled trial

Phase III: Postmarket Study
- Usually required to evaluate the long-term safety of the device
- Duration can be up to 5 years

Emergency Use of an Unapproved Medical Device

In situations where an IDE for the device does not exist, the proposed use is not approved under existing IDE, or the physician/institution is not approved under the IDE, the emergency use of unapproved device is allowed under the following circumstances:

1. The patient is in a life-threatening condition that needs immediate treatment.
2. No generally acceptable alternative for treating the patient is available.
3. The physician should get independent assessment by uninvolved physician.
4. An ICF was obtained from the patient or a legal representative.
5. The IRB was notified.
6. Authorization was obtained from the IDE holder, if an approved IDE for the device exists.

After an unapproved device is used in an emergency, the physician should:

1. Report to the IRB within 5 days of the emergency use.
2. Notify the sponsor.

The sponsor should notify the FDA immediately.

Compassionate Use of an Unapproved Medical Device

The compassionate use provision allows access for patients who do not meet the requirements for inclusion in the clinical investigation but for whom the treating physician believes the device may provide a benefit in treating and/or diagnosing their disease or condition. This provision is typically approved for individual patients but may be approved to treat a small group.

Criteria
  • Serious disease or condition
  • No therapeutic alternative
Time-frame   During clinical trial

FDA recognizes that there are circumstances in which an investigational device is the only option available for a patient faced with a serious, albeit not life-threatening, disease or condition. In these circumstances FDA uses its regulatory discretion in determining whether such use of an investigational device should occur. Prior FDA approval is needed before compassionate use occurs. In order to obtain the agency approval, the sponsor should submit an IDE supplement requesting approval for a protocol deviation under section 812.35(a) in order to treat the patient. The IDE supplement should include the following facts:

1. A description of the patient's condition and the circumstances necessitating treatment
2. A discussion of why alternatives therapies are unsatisfactory and why the probable risk of using the investigational device is no greater than the probable risk from the disease or condition
3. An identification of any deviations in the approved clinical protocol that may be needed in order to treat the patient
4. The patient protection measures that will be followed (informed consent, concurrence of IRB chairperson, clearance from the institution, independent assessment from uninvolved physician, authorization from IDE sponsor).

The physician should not treat the patient identified in the supplement until the FDA approves use of the device under the proposed circumstances. In reviewing this type of request, the FDA will consider the information above as well as whether the preliminary evidence of safety and effectiveness justifies such use and whether such use would interfere with the conduct of a clinical trial to support marketing approval.

If the request is approved, the attending physician should devise an appropriate schedule for monitoring the patient, taking into consideration the investigational nature of the device and the specific needs of the patient. The patient should be monitored to detect any possible problems arising from the use of the device. Compassionate use of the device requires a follow-up report to be submitted to FDA as an IDE supplement in which summary information regarding patient outcome is presented. If any problems occurred as a result of the device use, these should be reported in the supplement and to the reviewing IRB as soon as possible.

The compassionate use criteria and procedures can also be applied when a physician wishes to treat a few patients rather than an individual patient suffering from a serious disease or condition for which no alternative therapy adequately meets their medical need. In such a case the physician should request access to the investigational device through the IDE sponsor. The sponsor should submit an IDE supplement that includes the information identified above and indicates the number of patients to be treated. Such a supplement should describe the protocol to be followed or identify deviations from the approved clinical protocol. As with single-patient compassionate use, a monitoring schedule should be designed to meet the needs of the patients while recognizing the investigational nature of the device. Follow-up information on the use of the device should be submitted in an IDE supplement after all compassionate use patients have been treated.

FDA Acceptance of Foreign Clinical Studies[40]

FDA Views on Acceptance of Foreign Clinical Trials
- FDA cannot ensure the same level of human subject protection in foreign clinical trials as in domestic ones.
- Key entities overseeing or studying foreign research have raised concerns about foreign institutional review boards.

Recommendations for Sponsors of Foreign Clinical Trials
- Obtain information about the performance of foreign institutional review boards.
- Help foreign boards build capacity.
- Encourage greater sponsor monitoring.
- Encourage sponsors to obtain testimonies from foreign investigators.
- Develop a database to track the growth and location of foreign research.

In order for the FDA to accept foreign clinical studies not conducted under an IDE, IND, or non-IND foreign clinical studies as support for an IDE, IND, or application for marketing approval for a drug, biological product, or device, *the study must be conducted in accordance with good clinical practice (GCP)*, including review and approval by an independent ethics committee (IEC).

GCP is defined as a standard for the design, conduct, performance, monitoring, auditing, recording, analysis, and reporting of clinical trials in a way that provides assurance that the data and reported results are credible and accurate, and that the rights, safety, and well-being of trial subjects are protected. GCP also includes review and approval by an IEC before initiating a study, continuing IEC review of ongoing studies, and obtaining and documenting freely given informed consent of study subjects.

Global Clinical Studies

When global clinical studies at international sites are planned to be included in the study, the final clinical report is probably going to be submitted to the FDA as well as other international regulatory bodies.

So early communication is encouraged between US and international clinical teams to synchronize some of the the procedures of the study protocol and to make foreign regulations compatible with those the United States. The synchronization should extend to the reporting units of measurements in the CRFs, reporting of adverse events, and use of concomitant medications.

Differences may exist between the United States and other international sites in the reporting time periods of serious adverse events from the investigator to the sponsor or to regulatory authority. US regulations and the EU standard differ in their definition and wording regarding the seriousness or severity of an adverse event. EU regulations (EN 540) address adverse event seriousness based on the adverse event severity grading (mild, moderate, severe, and life threatening). The EU standard explains that a severe adverse event satisfies almost the same condition listed for a serious adverse event in an IDE study (causes death, hospitalization, prolonged hospitalization; requires intervention; results in a congenital anomaly or malignancy, or results in residual damage). The IDE regulations of the United States use the term *serious* as we defined above. To avoid differences in the definition of the seriousness of adverse events, sponsors should try to define adverse events based on seriousness as well as severity.

Also, to avoid confusion over the units of measurements used in the US with those used at international sites, alternatives for unit definitions could be provided or clinical sites instructed on which units that they should use in the study. Another example of synchronization of the clinical protocol procedures in global clinical trials is to use protocol concomitant medications. Because of economic or other reasons certain international sites can only use alternative drugs to those used in the United States. To avoid having numerous protocol deviations, the option of these alternative medications should be provided in the study protocol if it has no effect on the study's outcome (for more details on the global clinical studies, see Chapter 8).

In addition the US and the international clinical teams should coordinate their CRFs and provide a number of alternative unit definitions, or instruct investigators on which units to specifically use to avoid confusion among units. Because of the different system of units in Europe from the United States unit definitions and conversion should be made available at the sites or instructions on how to use specific units. Obvious examples are units of weight (defined in lb or kg), height (in or cm), and blood glucose (mg/dl or mM); other units should be specified if they are not defined by a single unit system. It is also important to reconcile differences in the definitions of certain adverse events and their reporting timelines in the United States compared with other international regions.

Finally, in device trials, center-to-center variations in a device's effect may be due to the physician's experience or training in using or implanting the device. Other explanations may include variations in patient population, patient management, and reporting practices. A scientifically credible explanation is required to account for variation of data across study centers. An analysis of variation in effects also becomes especially important when multicenter trials are conducted that include international sites, since any difference in data needs to be ascertained concerning the international sites' quality of health systems.

COMBINATION PRODUCTS

Combination products are products that include a drug or biologic with a device. Examples of these products are drug-eluting stents, drug delivery systems, hemostatic sealants, photodynamic therapy, gene therapy, and other such investigational treatments. Combination products are subjected to FDA review by a combined team of medical device and drug product reviewers at the FDA.

The sponsor of a combination product should be aware of the different clinical and scientific approaches at the FDA for devices and radiological Health (CDRH) from those used at the center for drug evaluation and research (CDER).

Key Differences between FDA Regulations in Device and Drug Development

Table 7.3 presents key differences between the FDA regulations regarding medical devices and drugs.

Combination Product Jurisdictional Determination— "Primary Mode of Action"

The FDA determines whether the combination product is a device, drug, or biologic mainly by the primary mode of action of the product. The following are examples of combination products that were determined to be devices, drugs, or biologics in accordance with the mode of action of the product.

Device
Drug-eluting stents
Insulin pump

TABLE 7.3   Key Differences between Device and Drug FDA Regulations

Criteria	Device	Drug
Rate of technology change	Rapid	Slow
Number of pivotal studies required for approval	1	2
Typical pivotal sample size	500–1,000	1,000–3,000
Reimbursement during the clinical trial	Frequent	Rare
Criteria for orphan status (treated patients/year)	4,000	200,000
Number of regulatory classes	3	1
Approval type	510(K), PMA	NDA, ANDA

Transdermal drug delivery patch
Implantable drug delivery
Pulmonary drug delivery
Photodynamic therapy

Drug
Liposome plus chemotherapy
AIDS protease inhibitor combination therapy

Biologic
Collagen plus antiproliferative agent

It should be noted that device designations are made by CDRH, drugs by CDER, and biologics by CBER. In most cases the same center will have the lead review and jurisdictional responsibility.

Because of the growing number of combination products, the FDA has established an office of combination products (OCP) to provide guidance to manufacturers pursuing development and market approval for combination products. In this capacity OCP also resolves jurisdictional and other issues that often arise during premarket review of combination products.

FDA Approval Process

The FDA approval of a combination product depends on the individual regulatory process of the drug and device components. A previous approval of the drug, even if approved for a different indication, makes it easier for approval to be obtained than for an investigational drug. For an investigational drug, CDER has to be satisfied regarding the safety of the drug. Drug-eluting stents provide a clear example of this process. The Taxus coronary stent manufactured by Boston Scientific

Corporation includes paclitaxel as the drug moiety in the combination product. Although this drug was approved earlier as anticancer agent, this approval facilitated the approval of the combination product because the drug's safety was established.

Pre-IDE/IND Submission

The sponsor should request a pre-IDE/IND meeting from the FDA. The following topics should be discussed in this meeting:

- Indication
- Potential benefit of the combination product
- Proposed FDA jurisdiction
- Preclinical testing
- Animal testing
- Proposed investigational plan for the clinical trial

The sponsor sends the meeting agenda, list of attendees, and list of questions. The FDA should respond to accept this meeting 4 to 6 weeks after receiving the meeting letter.

Pre-IDE/IND Meeting

After this meeting the sponsor should have good instructions from the FDA regarding:

- Confirmation of jurisdictional determination
- Preclinical testing requirements
- Device testing—mechanical, electrical
- Drug testing
  - Laboratory, CMC
  - Pharmacology, toxicology
- Animal studies
- Clinical trial design issues

Animal Studies

The main purpose of animal studies is to provide preliminary evidence of product safety to support initiation of a human clinical study. It is also advantageous if the sponsor can provide evidence for product effectiveness. The number of animals required, duration of the animal studies, and animal models used should be discussed with the FDA.

Pharmacokinetic (PK) Testing

Generation of PK data can be difficult for drug/device combination products because they often use very small drug doses. Accordingly a highly sensitive analytical assays for the drug needs to be developed.

When evaluating the PK studies, the FDA has particular interest in the development of an in vitro/in vivo correlation.

Dosing Studies in Animals

Although dosing studies are not formally required by FDA, they can be extremely important in addressing FDA concerns about how a particular therapeutic dose was established. It is useful to identify a low dose that was demonstrated to be subtherapeutic and high doses that proved to be toxic.

The FDA is interested in correlations between the in vitro or in vivo drug doses as compared to human doses.

Toxicity Testing

Evaluations of drug safety in animals at 1, 3, and 6 months usually are performed for a drug approved for a new indication. If the drug component is not already approved by the FDA, additional animal toxicity and human Phase I studies might be expected.

Bench Testing and Biocompatibility Testing

The sponsor must demonstrate that the drug and device do not chemically and/or physically adversely interact with each other. The sponsor must also determine the extent of particulate matter released from the combination product. Biocompatibility testing for blood-contacting implants typically includes determination of cytotoxicity, sensitization, acute toxicity, genotoxicity (mutagenecity), and hemocompatibility.

Clinical Trial Design

The preferred control group is an active control where patients are treated with a commercially available therapy. The alternative is a placebo control (i.e., sham therapy), which usually raises ethical and enrollment issues. The least attractive control group is a historical control based on objective performance criteria (OPC).

Key Information Resources

Key resources for combination products can be obtained from the Office of Combination Products (http://www.fda.gov/oc/combination) of the FDA, which also provides Draft Guidance for Industry: Combination Products, Timeliness of Premarket Reviews: Dispute Resolution Guidance (http://www.fda.gov/oc/combination/dispute.html).

STUDY COMMITTEES

Several study committees may be set up by the sponsor of the study prior to the initiation of the trial. Key examples are a Data Safety and Monitoring Board (DSMB), Clinical Events Committee (CEC), and Steering Committee. These study committees are contracted by the sponsor to evaluate and monitor safety issues in the study, adjudicate endpoints, review the scientific validity of the study's protocol, assess the study's quality and the scientific quality of the final study report. The oversight of these committees is important, particularly during pivotal studies in order to ensure the safety and effectiveness of the investigational device. The committees should be composed of members who are independent of the clinical study (with the exception of the Steering Committee). The main objectives of these study committees are as follows:

- To eliminate, or at least minimize, bias associated with the identification and assignment of serious adverse events or major adverse events through the use of a uniform procedure in identifying and defining these events.
- The DSMB has responsibility for reviewing the safety of clinical studies and can stop a clinical study if serious safety issues arise.
- The Steering Committee evaluates issues associated with the procedural aspects of the clinical trial (e.g., slow patient enrollment) and provides recommendations on their resolution.

Data Safety and Monitoring Board (DSMB)[41]

- Members of a data monitoring committee are experts external to the study that assess the progress, safety data, and the critical efficacy endpoints of the study, if needed.

- DSMB may review unblinded study information (on a patient level or treatment group level).
- Based on its review, the DSMB provides the sponsor with recommendations regarding study modification, continuation, or termination

Membership
- Membership is independent from participating investigators.
- Adequate representation should come from areas of clinical study conduct, biostatistics, bioethics, and therapeutics.
- The chair of the DSMB is selected from among the voting members.

Responsibilities of the DSMB
- Monitor patient safety through review of aggregate clinical study data and adverse events
- Adjudicate adverse events
- Act as an advisory panel on study design, study materials, study conduct, and patient safety issues
- Make recommendations for continuation, or early termination due to futility or safety concerns, early attainment of study objects, or protocol modifications

Meetings DSMB meetings are usually held annually but can be convened more frequently depending on the nature of the trial being monitored.

Recommendations from the DSMB DSMB gives its recommendation(s) to the trial principal investigator/project manager. If the DSMB recommends a study change for patient safety or efficacy, the trial project manager must implement the change as expeditiously as possible.

Clinical Events Committee (CEC)
- CECs are formed in clinical studies where endpoints are difficult to assess and include subjective components, or the study cannot be blinded.
- Members are clinical experts in a specific clinical area, charged with the responsibility of synchronizing and standardizing and the endpoint assessment.

- To allow for an unbiased endpoint assessment, the members of the committee are blinded to treatment assignment, whenever possible.
- CECs are widely used in the assessment of radiological endpoints.

Steering Committees

- This committee is usually created for large multicenter clinical trials.
- Members are appointed by the sponsor and are clinical experts not directly involved in the clinical trial, staff from the sponsor, and occasionally investigators.
- The Steering Committee often takes responsibility for the scientific integrity of a clinical trial, and also responsibility for the scientific validity of the study protocol, assessment of study's quality and conduct, as well as the scientific quality of the final study report.

FDA-SPONSOR MEETINGS

FDA Meetings with Study Sponsors

The FDA encourages different types of clinical study meetings with the industry sponsor of studies. These meetings can provide the following practical benefits to both the sponsors and the FDA:

1. Design testing and development plans that expedite review and approval
2. Savings of money and time
3. Collaborative actions
4. Minimal surprises

Before meeting with the FDA, the sponsor should think carefully about the desired outcomes and the agenda for the discussion. Also sponsor needs to be prepared to manage the meeting time effectively, bring qualified people to discuss focused questions, and never hesitate to ask for clarification. It should be further noted that if changes to device or protocol occur after the pre-IDE package has been submitted, a meeting could be canceled or postponed. The sponsor should realize that guarantees or binding commitments do not result from meetings, unless the meeting is conducted to bring a determination or agreement on an issue. Studies or devices do not get approved at these meetings.

Timing of Meetings

Meetings may be held at any point in the *premarket phase*:

- Prior to conducting "proof of concept" animal studies
- Preclinical
- Prior to expanding clinical trials from feasibility to pivotal phase
- Pre-PMA
- During the PMA submission: day 100 PMA meetings
- Postdeficiency letter for 510(K) or PMA
- Appeal a final decision on a PMA or 510(K) or an IDE disapproval
- Agreement or determination meeting

Prior to Proof of Concept   Face-to-face meetings are usually not held at this stage (premature).

- Discuss concepts, broad outline of test plan, bench test methodologies (e.g., use of consensus standards, need for animal studies, need for clinical studies)
- Discuss possible regulatory pathways for device approval
- Discuss potential combination product issues

Preclinical Phase   Pre-IDE meetings/teleconferences are encouraged at this stage.

- Prototype evaluated in preliminary animal models
- Proposed clinical application (but not specific patient population) and indication for use
- FDA feedback on:
  - Bench testing plan—methods, standards
  - Animal study protocols
  - Feasibility study protocols
  - Preliminary guidance on SR/NSR (need for IDE)

- Preliminary (nonbinding) guidance on regulatory pathway
- Feedback dependent on focused questions

Pre-IDE meetings are intended for:

- Tool to provide informal feedback on:
  - Preclinical test plan
  - Clinical/statistical test plan
  - Nonsignificant risk (NSR)/exempt investigations
  - Out of the US (OUS) investigations
- NOT intended to be:
  - A tool for negotiation
  - An iterative process
  - Modular review
  - Review of data ("pre-510(K)," "pre-PMA")
  - As in depth as an IDE or marketing application review
  - Legally binding
  - Method for dispute resolution

Prior to Initiating Pivotal Trials   Meetings/teleconferences with FDA are encouraged at this stage.

- Feasibility studies completed (or nearly completed)
- Device design finalized
- Animal studies completed (or in follow-up)
- Pivotal trial protocol synopsis (primary and secondary endpoints, duration, evaluation methods, statistical analysis)
- Specific indication for use (and patient population) determination
- FDA will give feedback on:
  - Need for more bench/animal studies
  - Need for pilot study prior to initiating pivotal study
  - Proposed pivotal study protocol: endpoints, duration, evaluation, statistical analysis plan
  - Proposed regulatory pathway
  - Proposed indication for use
  - Preliminary nonbinding feedback on expedited status, need for advisory panel meeting
- Feedback dependent on focused questions

Scheduling Informal Pre-IDE Meetings

These meetings are not determined or agreed-upon in advance.

- Planning/scheduling may be done by project manager (usually 3–4 weeks after pre-IDE received)
- Complete pre-meeting package needed before meeting will be scheduled
- Meetings subject to cancellation or postponement if extensive new information is submitted after the meeting has been scheduled

Meeting Preparation

Complete Package Must Be Submitted in Advance   The FDA must have the complete pre-meeting package in order to schedule a meeting. The package must be:

- Received by branch chief; review team determined
- Assigned to lead reviewer
- Copies prepared (or requested) and distributed
- Internal pre-meeting/sponsor meeting scheduled
- Team members review package, prepare memos prior to pre-meeting
- Internal pre-meeting held to discuss issues, reach consensus, and obtain progress information from team/management

Agenda and Attendee List   Sponsors are responsible for preparing and sending the agenda to the FDA. Your time and the FDA's time is valuable—make the most of it. Preparation should include:

- Time allocated to each topic
- Maximized time for discussion of issues that need to be clarified by the FDA
- Time that the meeting will begin and end (typically no more than 1–1.5 hours)
- List of attendees (and their affiliations) submitted in advance
- Sign-in sheet to be circulated during meeting, copied, and provided to the sponsor

Focused Questions   During the internal pre-meeting, the FDA team discusses deficiencies and other issues. The meeting centers on discussing focused questions provided by sponsor:

- On efficient use of resources
- On any pressing matters about the clinical protocol not get addressed
- Any other specifies about the proposed clinical studies

Meeting Minutes   After the FDA-sponsor meeting, the FDA sometimes asks the sponsor to complete meeting minutes and send it to the FDA for review and confirmation.

REGISTRATION OF CLINICAL TRIALS[42,43]

ClinicalTrials.gov, a federally sponsored website, provides a comprehensive listing of federally and privately supported clinical studies. Through the information provided on this website, clinical trials investigating a wide range of diseases and conditions can be found.

ClinicalTrials.gov was initiated as a result of the Food and Drug Administration Modernization Act of November 1997. The legislation requires the Department of Health and Human Services, through the NIH, to establish a registry of clinical trials for both federally and privately funded trials "of experimental treatments for serious or life-threatening diseases or conditions."

Each record provided in *ClinicalTrials.gov* lists the following:

- Disease or condition and experimental treatments studied
- Title, description, and design of study, including the purpose of study and eligibility criteria
- Requirements for participation
- Study site location and contact information
- Links to relevant information at other health websites, such MedlinePlus and PubMed

Since scientists tend to publish their positive findings more often than any negative findings (publication bias), it has become common practice in the medical device industry to register clinical trials at *ClinicalTrials.gov*. A comprehensive registry of initiated clinical trials, with each trial assigned a unique identifier, should provide reviewers, physicians, and others (e.g., consumers) with important information about ongoing trials.

IMPLEMENTATION OF THE HIPAA PRIVACY RULE
IN CLINICAL RESEARCH

The privacy provisions of the federal law, the Health Insurance Portability and Accountability Act of 1996 (HIPAA), apply to health information created or maintained by health care providers who engage in certain electronic transactions, health plans, and health care clearing houses. The Office for Civil Rights (OCR) is the departmental component responsible for implementing and enforcing the privacy regulation.

Who Must Comply with the New HIPAA Privacy Standards?

Health care providers who conduct certain financial and administrative transactions electronically must comply with the HIPAA privacy standards.

What Does the HIPAA Privacy Rule Do?

The HIPAA privacy rule creates national standards to protect individuals' medical records and other personal health information. The privacy regulations govern a provider's use and disclosure of health information and grant individuals new rights of access and control. The regulations also establish civil and criminal penalties for violations of patient privacy.

Covered Entities
- Health plans
- Health care clearing houses
- Health care providers who conduct electronic transactions related to third-party billing

Protected Health Information (PHI)
- Relates to past, present, or future health, or health care, or payment for health care
- Identifies the individual, directly or indirectly

PHI can be written, electronic, or verbal. Examples include clinic charts, billing records, rounding lists, medical media, clinic or research databases, and hallway conversations.

When Does HIPAA Apply to Research?

The rules apply if PHI is accessed to initiate the study or created during the study.

Allowable Conditions for Use of PHI in Research

Obtain written authorization from the patient, or meet one of the following criteria:

- De-identified data
- IRB waiver of individual authorization
- Limited data set plus data use agreement
- Activities that are "preparatory to research"
- Research on decedents

Conditions Not Requiring Authorization
- De-identified data
- Waiver of authorization by an IRB or privacy board
- Limited data sets
- Activities that are "preparatory to research"
- Research on decedents

Revised IRB Waiver Criteria
- Use or disclosure poses minimal risk to patient privacy
- Research could not be done without the waiver
- Research could not be done without PHI
- Risks are reasonable compared to benefits
- Plan to protect identifiers from improper use and disclosure
- Plan to destroy identifiers at the appropriate time
- Assurances from the PI that the PHI will not be reused

Required Elements for Authorizations
- A specific description of the purpose of the authorization and the information to be used or disclosed
- The names or classes of individuals authorized to make the use or disclosure
- The names or classes of individuals authorized to receive the use or disclosure
- An expiration date for the authorization

- A statement that the individual has a right to revoke the authorization
- The consequences of refusal to sign
- A statement that the information used or disclosed pursuant to the authorization may be subject to re-disclosure and no longer protected by the Privacy Rule.

What Makes It PHI? Health Information plus Identifying Elements
- Names
- Street address, city, county, precinct, zip code
- Dates (e.g., DOB, DOD, admission, discharge, procedure dates)
- Ages over 89
- Phone and numbers
- Fax numbers
- Email addresses
- Social security numbers
- Medical record number
- Health plan numbers
- Account numbers
- Certificate/license numbers
- License plate number
- Device identifiers and serial numbers
- Internet protocol (IP) address
- Biometric identifiers, including finger and voice prints
- Full face photographic images and any comparable images
- Any other unique identifying number, characteristic, or code

De-identified Data
- All 18 identifiers must be removed.
- Data with removed identitie's are not necessarily designed for research purposes.
- If the researcher is accessing or receiving only de-identified data for a project, HIPAA rules do not apply.

Limited Data Sets (LDS)
- LDS are a category of PHI that excludes specific readily identifiable information—16 identifiers must be excluded—and can be used for research purposes.

- To use or disclose a LDS for research, public health, or health care operations, the recipient must enter into a Data Use Agreement.
- Disclosures of PHI per an LDS need not be included in an accounting for disclosures.

Limited data sets may not include:

- Names
- Street addresses
- Telephone and fax numbers
- Email addresses
- SSNs
- Certificate or license numbers
- Vehicle ID or serial numbers
- Full face photos or comparable images
- MR numbers
- Health plan beneficiary numbers
- Biometric identifiers

Limited data sets may include:

- Admission dates
- Birth dates
- Discharge dates
- Service dates
- Death date
- Age
- Zip code (all digits)
- Gender

Waiver of the Authorization Requirement

- Examples: Retrospective chart review
- Accessing medical records to screen subjects for a clinical trial
- Application for waiver must be approved by an IRB or Privacy Board
- Use and disclosure poses no more than minimal risk to privacy:
  - Adequate data protection plan
  - Adequate plan to destroy identifiers
  - Adequate assurances against re-use or disclosure

- Research is not practicable without waiver
- Research is not practicable without PHI

Preparatory to Research
- Example: Reviewing medical records to determine adequacy of patient baseline information
- For the PHI viewed, only de-identified data can be **recorded**.
- Covered entity must obtain an attestation from the researcher:
  - Review of PHI is solely to prepare a protocol or formulate hypotheses.
  - PHI will not be removed from the covered entity.
  - PHI being reviewed is necessary for research purposes.
- This activity generally precedes HSC application, if there is no formal protocol developed.

Recruitment Questions
- Are you using PHI to identify subjects?
- If so, what permissions do you need to gain access to the PHI?
- Do you have a treatment relationship with the prospective subject?

Allowable Recruitment Practices
- Providers can always talk to their own patients about studies they are conducting.
- Providers can notify the patient that they might qualify for a particular study, and the patient can initiate the contact with the researcher.
- The provider or the medical records department can release information to researchers if:
  - The patient signs a pre-approved authorization so that the provider can give PHI to researcher, or
  - The IRB approves a partial waiver of authorization for recruitment purposes. (The HIPAA waiver criteria must be met.) The researcher identifies the subjects, and a member of the treatment team makes the initial contact.
- Patients can self-refer from ads, flyers, and other public postings.

Subjects' Access to Research Records
- Patients have right to access their "designated record set"—the set of medical and billing records that are used to make decisions about them.

- Any temporary denial of access must be accepted by the patient.
- Research records generally are not part of the designated record set.
- Any clinically relevant information must be put into the medical record.

INSTITUTIONAL REVIEW BOARDS (IRB)

The regulations pertaining to IRB membership, functions and responsibilities can be found in 21 CFR Part 56 and 45 CFR Part 46. The functions and responsibilities of the IRB are discussed in Chapter 2 in the "Development of Clinical Protocols, Case Report Forms, Clinical Standard Operating Procedures, Informed Consent Form, Study Regulatory Binder, and Other Clinical Materials" section under "Quality Assurance and Data Collection."

IRB Structure and Function

IRB Structure In accordance with FDA regulations, an IRB is designated to review and monitor clinical research involving human subjects. An IRB has the authority to approve, request modifications, or disapprove clinical research proposals. The purpose of the IRB review is to ensure that appropriate steps are taken to protect the rights and welfare of humans participating as subjects in clinical research. This is usually done prior to initiating the research and by periodic review during the conduct of the research. Although institutions engaged in research involving human subjects will usually have their own IRBs (local IRB) to oversee research conducted within the institution or by the staff of the institution, FDA regulations permit an institution without an IRB to arrange for an outside IRB (central IRB) to be responsible for initial and continuing review of studies conducted at the non-IRB institution. It should be noted that IRBs can agree to review research from affiliated or unaffiliated investigators. If the IRB routinely conducts these reviews, the IRB policies should authorize such reviews and the process should be described in the IRB's written procedures. A hospital IRB may review outside studies on an individual basis when it has the specific information about the research to be conducted. The main purpose of the IRB function is the review of the informed's consent (IC) to ensure the rights and welfare of participating subjects. The review of the IC may include the documentation of the institution's compliance with applicable regulations and institution policy. In accordance with the FDA regulations, for research involving more than minimal risk, study subjects should be informed whether any compensation and any medical treatment(s) are available if injury occurs, and if so, what the injuries are, or where further information may be obtained. Any statement that compensation is not offered must avoid waiving or appearing to waive any of the subject's rights or releasing or appearing to release the investigator, sponsor, or institution from liability for negligence.

IRBs should include membership that has a diversity of representative capacities and disciplines. The FDA regulations require that as part of being qualified as an IRB member, the IRB must have diversity of members, including consideration of race, gender, cultural backgrounds, and sensitivity to such issues as community attitudes. For example, one member could be otherwise unaffiliated with the institution and have a primary concern in a nonscientific area. The use of formally appointed alternate IRB members is acceptable to the FDA, provided that the IRB's written procedures describe the appointment and function of alternate members. The IRB roster should identify the primary member(s) for whom each alternate member may substitute. To ensure maintaining an appropriate quorum, the alternate's qualifications should be comparable to the primary member to be replaced. The IRB minutes should document when an alternate member replaces a primary member. FDA regulations require at least one member of the IRB to have primary concerns in the scientific area and at least one to have primary concerns in the nonscientific area. Most IRBs include physicians and PhD-level physical or biological scientists. Such members satisfy the requirement for at least one scientist. In accordance with the FDA regulations, when an IRB encounters studies involving science beyond the expertise of the members, the IRB may use a consultant to assist in the review. Lawyers, clergy, and ethicists have been cited as examples of persons whose primary concerns would be in nonscientific areas. Some members have training in both scientific and nonscientific disciplines, such as a JD, or an RN. While these members are of great value to an IRB, other members who are unambiguously nonscientific should be appointed to satisfy the nonscientist requirement. When selecting IRB members, the potential for conflicts of interest should be considered because the FDA regulations prohibit any member from participating in the IRB's initial or continuing review of any study in which the member has a conflicting interest, except to provide information requested by the IRB. When members frequently have conflicts and must absent themselves from deliberation and abstain from voting, their contributions to the group review process may be diminished and can hinder the review procedure.

IRB Procedures

Expedited Review   Certain kinds of research may be reviewed and approved without convening a meeting of the entire IRB members. The FDA regulations permit an IRB to review certain categories of research through an expedited procedure if the research involves no more than minimal risk. The IRB may also use the expedited review procedure to review minor changes in previously approved research during the period covered by the original approval. Under an expedited review procedure, review of research may be carried out by the IRB chairperson or by one or more experienced members of the IRB designated by the chairperson. The reviewer(s) may exercise all the authorities of the IRB, except disapproval. Research may only be disapproved following review by the full committee. The FDA regulations do not require public or sponsor access to IRB records. However, FDA does not prohibit the sponsor from requesting IRB records. The IRB and the institution may establish a policy on whether minutes or a pertinent portion of the minutes are provided to sponsors. Because of variability, each IRB also needs to be aware of state and local laws regarding access to IRB records.

Review of Risks   For studies conducted under an investigational new drug application (NDA), or an investigational device exemption (IDE), FDA regulations outline the criteria for IRB approval of research. The IRB should ensure that the risks to subjects are minimized and that the risks to subjects are reasonable in relation to the anticipated benefits. The risks cannot be adequately evaluated without review of the results of previous animal and human studies.

Review of Emergency Use of a Test Article   FDA regulations allow for one emergency use of a test article in an institution without prospective IRB review, provided that such emergency use is reported to the IRB within five working days after such use. An emergency use is defined as a single use (or single course of treatment, e.g., the use of a medical device in life-threatening condition) with one subject. "Subsequent use" would be a second use with that subject or the use with another subject. In its review of the emergency use, if it is anticipated that the test article may be used again, the IRB should request a protocol and consent document(s) be developed so that an approved protocol would be in place when the next need arises. Despite the best efforts of the clinical investigator and the IRB, a situation may occur where a second emergency use needs to be considered. FDA believes it is inappropriate to deny emergency treatment to an individual when the only obstacle is lack of time for the IRB to convene, review the use, and give approval. IRBs are required to function under written procedures. One of these procedural requirements requires ensuring "prompt reporting to the IRB of changes in a research activity." The completion of the study is a change in activity and should be reported to the IRB. For more on such emergency use, see the section under "Emergency Use of a Medical Device" in Chapter 7.

Monitoring of Clinical Research   FDA does not expect IRBs to routinely observe consent interviews, observe the conduct of the study, or review study records. However, FDA regulations give the IRB the authority to observe, or have a third-party observe, the consent process and the research. When and if the IRB is concerned about the conduct of the study or the process for obtaining consent, the IRB may consider whether, as part of providing adequate oversight of the study, an active audit is warranted.

Communications of Investigators and Sponsors with the IRB   Clinical investigators should report adverse events directly to the responsible IRB, and should send progress reports directly to that IRB. FDA does require direct communication between the sponsors and the IRBs. However, FDA does not prohibit direct communication between the sponsor and the IRB, and recognizes that doing so could result in more efficient resolution of some problems.

Submission of a Study to a Second IRB   When an IRB disapproves a study, it must provide a written statement of the reasons for its decision to the investigator and the institution. If the study is submitted to a second IRB, a copy of this written statement should be included with the study's documentation so that it can make an informed decision about the study. All pertinent information about the study should be provided to the second IRB.

Inspections of IRB   The Division of Scientific Investigations, Center for Drug Evaluation and Research, maintains an inventory of the IRBs that have been inspected, including dates of inspection and classification. The Division recently began including the results of inspections assigned by the Center for Biologics Evaluation and Research and the Center for Devices and Radiological Health. This information is available through Freedom of Information Act (FOIA) procedures. Once an investigational file has been closed, the correspondence between

FDA and the IRB and the narrative inspectional report are also available under FOI.

IRB Records   When an IRB approves a study, continuing review should be performed at least annually. All of the records listed in FDA regulations are required to be maintained. The clock starts on the date of approval, whether or not subjects have been enrolled. Written progress reports should be received from the clinical investigator for all studies that are in approved status prior to the date of expiration of IRB approval. If subjects were never enrolled, the clinical investigator's progress report would indicate this. Such studies may receive continuing IRB review using expedited procedures. If the study is finally canceled without subject enrollment, records should be maintained for at least three years after the cancellation.

Subjects' Informed Consent   Many clinical investigators use the consent document as a guide for the verbal explanation of the study. The subject's signature provides documentation of agreement to participate in a study but is only one part of the consent process. The entire informed consent process involves giving a subject adequate information concerning the study, providing adequate opportunity for the subject to consider all options, responding to the subject's questions, ensuring that the subject has comprehended this information, obtaining the subject's voluntary agreement to participate, and continuing to provide information as the subject or situation requires. To be effective, the process should provide ample opportunity for the investigator and the subject to exchange information and ask questions. It is acceptable to send the informed consent document to the legally authorized representative by facsimile and conduct the consent interview by telephone when the legally authorized representative can read the consent as it is discussed. If the legally authorized representative agrees, he/she can sign the consent and return the signed document to the clinical investigator by facsimile.

The regulation require a copy of the IRB-approved document that was given to the subject to obtain consent. One purpose of providing the person signing the form with a copy of the consent document is to allow the subject to review the information with others, both before and after making a decision to participate in the study, as well as providing a continuing reference for items such as scheduling of procedures and emergency contacts.

FDA does not require any subject to "waive" a legal right. Rather, FDA requires that subjects be informed that complete privacy does not apply in the context of research involving FDA-regulated products. Under the authority of the Federal Food, Drug, and Cosmetic Act, FDA may inspect and copy clinical records to verify information submitted by a sponsor. FDA generally will not copy a subject's name during the inspection unless a more detailed study of the case is required or there is reason to believe that the records do not represent the actual cases studied or results obtained. The consent document should not state or imply that FDA needs clearance or permission from the clinical investigator, the subject, or the IRB for such access. When clinical investigators conduct studies for submission to FDA, they agree to allow FDA access to the study records, as outlined in FDA regulations. Informed consent documents should make it clear that, by participating in research, the subject's records automatically become part of the research database. Subjects do not have the option to keep their records from being audited/reviewed by FDA. When an individually identifiable medical record (usually kept by the clinical investigator, not by the IRB) is copied and reviewed by the Agency, proper confidentiality procedures are followed within FDA. Consistent with laws relating to public disclosure of information and the law enforcement responsibilities of the Agency, however, absolute confidentiality cannot be guaranteed. FDA does not require a third person to witness the consent interview unless the subject or representative is not given the opportunity to read the consent document before it is signed.

The person who conducts the consent interview should be knowledgeable about the study and able to answer questions. FDA does not specify who this individual should be. Some sponsors and some IRBs require the clinical investigator to personally conduct the consent interview. However, if someone other than the clinical investigator conducts the interview and obtains consent, this responsibility should be formally delegated by the clinical investigator and the person so delegated should have received appropriate training to perform this activity. Illiterate persons who understand English may have the consent read to them and "make their mark," if appropriate under applicable state law. FDA requirements for signature of a witness to the consent process and signature of the person conducting consent interview must be followed if a "short form" is used. Clinical investigators should be cautious when enrolling subjects who may not truly understand what they have agreed to do. The IRB should consider illiterate persons as likely to be vulnerable to coercion and undue influence and should determine that appropriate additional safeguards are in place when enrollment of such persons is anticipated. FDA does not require the signature of a witness when the subject reads and is capable of understanding the consent document, as outlined in FDA regulations. The intended purpose is to have the witness present during the entire consent interview and to attest to the accuracy of the presentation and the apparent understanding of the subject. If the intent of the regulation were only to attest to the validity of the subject's signature, witnessing would also be required when the subject reads the consent.

The sponsor usually provides a service to the clinical investigator and the IRB when it prepares suggested study-specific wording for the scientific and technical content of the consent document. However, the IRB has the responsibility and authority to determine the adequacy and appropriateness of all of the wording in the consent. If an IRB insists on wording the sponsor cannot accept, the sponsor may decide not to conduct the study at that site.

For medical device studies that are conducted under an IDE, copies of all forms and informational materials to be provided to subjects to obtain informed consent must be submitted to FDA as part of the IDE. For investigational devices, the informed consent is a required part of the IDE submission. It is therefore approved by FDA as part of the IDE application. When an IRB makes substantive changes in the document, FDA re-approval is required, and the sponsor is necessarily involved in this process. FDA regulations for other products do not specifically require the sponsor to review IRB-approved consent documents. However, most sponsors do conduct such reviews to ensure that the wording is acceptable to the sponsor. Protocol amendments must receive IRB review and approval before they are implemented, unless an immediate change is necessary to eliminate an apparent hazard to the subjects. Those subjects who are presently enrolled and actively participating in the study should be informed of the change if it might relate to the subjects' willingness to continue their participation in the study. FDA does not require re-consenting of subjects that have completed their active participation in the study, or of subjects who are still actively participating when the change will not affect their participation, for example, when the change will be implemented only for subsequently enrolled subjects.

Informed Consent Document Content   The FDA requirements for informed consent are the minimum basic elements of informed consent that must be presented to a research subject. An IRB may require inclusion of any additional information that it considers important to a subject's decision to participate in a research study. FDA requires contacts for questions about the research, the research subject's rights, and in case of a research-related injury. It does not specify whom to contact. The same person may be listed for all three. However, FDA and most IRBs believe it is better to name a knowledgeable person other than the clinical investigator as the contact for study subject rights. Having the clinical investigator as the only contact may inhibit subjects from reporting concerns and/or possible abuses.

Clinical Investigations   The FDA regulations require IRB review and approval of regulated clinical investigations, whether or not the study involves institutionalized subjects. FDA has included noninstitutionalized subjects because it is inappropriate to apply a double standard for the protection of research subjects based on whether or not they are institutionalized.

An investigator may be able to obtain IRB review by submitting the research proposal to a community hospital, a university/medical school, an independent IRB, a local or state government health agency, or other organizations. If IRB review cannot be accomplished by one of these means, investigators may contact the FDA for assistance.

Treatment IND/IDE   Test articles given to human subjects under a treatment IND/IDE require prior IRB approval, with two exceptions. If a life-threatening emergency exists, as defined by FDA regulations, exemptions from IRB requirement may be followed. In addition FDA may grant the sponsor or sponsor/investigator a waiver of the IRB requirement. An IRB may still choose to review a study even if FDA has granted a waiver.

IRB letters to study sponsors must contain the following information:

- Date of the IRB meeting
- What is being reviewed
  - Initial approval
  - Annual approval
  - Protocol amendment to include the amendment number
  - Adverse event
  - Safety report
- Whether the protocol is "approved"
  - If the IRB required modifications, the letter must state that the protocol is approved, contingent on changes or modifications.
  - After changes or modifications are completed, as required by the IRB, the IRB chairperson may do an expedited review of the changes. This expedited review is at the discretion of the IRB.

- The type of review
  - Expedited approval
  - Full board approval

The sponsor of the study must maintain copies of all reports submitted to the IRB and reports of all actions by the IRB:

- Prior approval
- Protocol
- Modifications to the protocol/amendments, addenda
- Subject consent
- Patient/subject recruitment materials
- Investigator brochure
- All correspondence

Types of Reviews (21 CFR 56 and 45 CFR 46)

Three types of serious are conducted by the reviewing IRB:

- Full review
- Expedited review
- Exempt review

Full Review   When is a full board approval required?

- First time approval
- Active studies with patients on treatment
- If there is a risk involved (increased risk or additional risk)
- Change in treatment
- Amendment with more than minimum risk

Expedited Review
- Minimal risk
- Minor changes in previously approved research

Generally, if study is closed to group accrual, or no patients are on treatment, an annual review can be approved by expedited review.

- Reason for expedited review must be noted on approval.
- The IRB always has the right to require full board approval.

Exempt Review   Some examples are collection of blood samples from healthy/nonpregnant adults, sputum, nail clippings, and other non-invasive procedures.

Office for Human Research Protections (OHRP)

Common OHRP Findings of IRB Noncompliance Issues

Initial and Continuing Review
   • Research conducted without IRB review
   • Failure of IRB to review HHS grant applications
   • IRB lacks sufficient information to make determinations required for approval of research
   • Inadequate IRB review at convened meetings
   • Inadequate continuing review
   • Contingent approval of research with substantive changes and no additional review by the convened IRB
   • Failure to conduct continuing review at least once per year
   • IRB meeting convened without quorum (nonscientist absent)
   • IRB meeting convened without quorum (lack of a majority)
   • IRB members with conflicting interest participated in IRB review of research

Expedited Review Procedures
   • Inappropriate use of expedited review procedures for initial or continuing IRB review
   • Inappropriate use of expedited review procedures for review of protocol changes
   • Failure to advise IRB members of expedited approvals

Reporting of Unanticipated Problems and IRB Review of Protocol Changes
   • Failure to report unanticipated problems to IRB, institutional officials, and OHRP
   • Failure of IRB to review protocol changes
   • Inadequate IRB review of protocol changes

Informed Consent
   • Failure to obtain legally effective informed consent
   • Failure to document informed consent

- Deficient informed consent documents (ICDs) in general
- Inadequate ICD for specific research/lack of required elements
- Inadequate ICD for specific research/lack of additional elements
- ICD language too complex
- Exculpatory language in ICDs
- Standard surgical consent documents lacking required elements of informed consent
- Inappropriate boiler plate ICDs
- Enrollment procedures not minimizing possibility of coercion or undue influence

IRB Membership, Expertise, Staff, Support, and Workload
- Lack of diversity of IRB membership
- Lack of IRB expertise on research involving children
- Lack of prisoner/prisoner representative for IRB review of research involving prisoners
- Conflict resulting from office of research support (sponsored programs) serving as a voting
- Member of the IRB
- IRB chair and members lacking sufficient understanding of HHS regulations
- Designation of an additional IRB without prior OHRP approval
- Inadequate IRB resources
- Overburdened IRB

Documentation of IRB Activities, Findings, and Procedures
- Inadequate IRB records
- Inadequate IRB minutes
- Poorly maintained IRB files
- Failure of IRB to determine that criteria for IRB approval are satisfied
- Failure of IRB to document consideration of additional safeguards for vulnerable subjects
- Failure of IRB to make required findings when reviewing research involving children
- Failure of IRB to make required findings when reviewing research involving prisoners
- Failure of IRB to make and document required findings for waiver of informed consent

- Failure to make required findings for IRB waiver of a signed informed consent document
- Lack of appropriate written IRB policies and procedures
- Inadequate procedures for oversight of repository activities
- Inadequate procedure for reporting and review of unanticipated problems

FDA'S OVERSIGHT OF CLINICAL TRIALS (BIORESEARCH MONITORING)

The FDA program of on-site inspections for GCP and GLP is the Bioresearch Monitoring Program (BIMO). Inspections may be conducted anywhere in the world for studies submitted to FDA. This program includes inspections of:

- Clinical investigators
- Sponsors, monitors, CROs
- Institutional review boards
- Bioequivalence laboratories and facilities
- GLP facilities (nonclinical studies)

Data auditing is a major component of GCP- BIMO inspections conducted at clinical investigator and sponsor sites, whereas IRB inspections are more oriented toward the process of IRB review and the maintenance of required records.

Program Objectives

The BIMO program has two main objectives:

- To verify the quality and integrity of bioresearch data
- To protect the rights and welfare of human research subjects

Inspection of Clinical Investigators

Study-specific inspections are provided as well as audits of physicians, veterinarians, and other investigators conducting clinical trials of human and veterinary drugs, medical devices, biologicals, and so forth. The primary regulatory obligations of clinical investigators can be summarized as follows:

- Follow the approved protocol or research plan.
- Obtain informed consent and adhere to FDA regulations regarding protection of human research subjects.
- Maintain adequate and accurate records of study data.
- Administer test articles only to subjects under control of the investigator.

Study specific data audits are announced in advance. Inspection includes an interview with the clinical investigator and an in-depth data audit to validate study findings and verify the investigator's compliance with regulations. The FDA BIMO audit is usually performed for every NDA and PMA, or it may be assigned based on complaints received by FDA (from subjects, IRBs, industry).

Compliance Classifications   The outcome of the BIMO audit could be summarized as follows:

No Action Indicated   No objectionable conditions or practices were found during the inspection (or the objectionable conditions found do not justify further regulatory action).

Voluntary Action Indicated   Objectionable conditions or practices were found, but FDA is not prepared to take or recommend any administrative or regulatory action.

Official Action Indicated
- Regulatory and/or administrative actions are recommended because of significant objectionable observations.
- Warning letters and other correspondence are initiated.

Regulatory Obligations of Sponsors
- Label investigational products appropriately
- Initiate, withhold, or discontinue clinical trials as required
- Refrain from commercialization of investigational products
- Control the distribution and return of investigational products
- Select qualified investigators to conduct and monitor studies
- Disseminate appropriate information to investigators
- Evaluate and report adverse experiences
- Maintain adequate records of studies
- Submit progress reports and the final results of studies

Inspection of Study Sponsors

- Study-specific inspections routinely announced in advance, consisting of records' audit and interviews, with the inspection assigned for each PMA in CDRH
- Objective is to evaluate compliance with regulations and validate data
- Principal areas covered:
  - Organization and personnel
  - Selection of clinical investigators
  - Selection of monitors and monitoring procedures
  - Reporting of adverse experiences and reactions
  - Test article characterization and accountability

Preparation for an FDA Audit

The preparation of the FDA audit requires that people involved in this process be highly organized and have a clear understanding of the deliverables that the inspector may request. The general preparation of the FDA inspection includes the preparation of documents such as personnel CVs, job descriptions, organizational charts, and SOPs. The inspector may request special CRFs or specific reporting data on adverse event reports, safety and effectiveness data, device accountability, monitoring reports, and so forth. It is important that the person who is handling the inspector's request deliver the specific requested items in a timely manner and be prepared to respond to the inspector's questions and comments.

Regulatory/Administrative Follow-up with BIMO Audit Outcome

If the above-listed outcomes of a BIMO audit are not addressed satisfactorily, the following sanctions could be imposed on the sponsor or the reviewing IRB:

- Rejection of study
- Disqualification
- Prosecution
- Restriction of IRB approval of new studies or entry of subjects
- Disqualification of IRB

Common Deficiencies Cited by the FDA

- Failure to adequately monitor study
- Failure to document monitoring visits

- Failure to have or follow SOPs
- Failure to maintain product accountability records
- Failure to select qualified monitors

CODE OF FEDERAL REGULATIONS OF MEDICAL DEVICES

US Code 21 (h) Food, Drug, and Cosmetic Act. Web Address: http://www.fda.gove/opacom/laws/fdcact/fdcact1.htm. The 21 CFR Regulating medical devices are as follows:

Part 812—Investigational Device Exemptions
Part 814—Premarket Approval of Medical Devices
Part 803—Medical Device Reporting
Part 860—Medical Device Classification Procedures
Part 50-ICF

21 CFR 50.25—Elements of ICF—

Part 56—IRB
Part 11—Electronic Records

8

DESIGN ISSUES IN MEDICAL DEVICES STUDIES

Design, Execution, and Management of Medical Device Clinical Trials,
by Salah Abdel-aleem
Copyright © 2009 John Wiley & Sons, Inc.

This chapter addresses clinical trial issues that could prove challenging, such as the choice of the study control group, methods of assigning intervention, masking, and superiority or noninferiority study design. This chapter also discusses some important components of the final clinical report that are often not reported properly, such as examination of data across study sites and repeated measurements (see also Chapter 6). Since the selection of the historic control remains to be one of the most challenging issues in medical device clinical trials, an entire section was devoted to this subject in this chapter, with the data from two recent PMA studies used as examples of how the FDA is reviewing and approving this type of trials.

DESIGN OF THE CLINICAL TRIAL[44]

In designing the clinical study, the following parameters of the trial should be clearly addressed:

- The trial objective
- Pilot or feasibility study
- Identification and selection of variables
- Study population
- Control population
- Methods of assigning interventions
- Specific trial designs
- Masking
- Trial site and investigator
- Sample size and statistical power

ASSUMPTIONS AND PARAMETERS OF CLINICAL TRIAL DESIGN

The Trial Objective (The Research Question)

The following questions should be answered clearly when designing the main objective of the trial:

- What is the proper way to evaluate effectiveness in the target condition and population?
- What are the unique safety concerns of the device intervention?

- Is the device as effective as, or more effective than, another intervention? If so, is it as safe or safer?
- Is the evaluation of safety and effectiveness limited to a particular subgroup of patients?
- What is the best clinical measure of safety and effectiveness?

Pilot or Feasibility Study

Pilot or feasibility studies are designed to achieve the following:

- A limited trial to test a theory or new technique, but the pilot study should not be too broad (i.e., a "fishing expedition")
- A number of issues related to the clinical trial that can be refined, including device use, patient processing and monitoring, data gathering and validation, and physician capabilities and concerns
- Care taken to refine the measurements of critical variables, including potential outcome variables and influencing variables including potential sources of bias

Identification and Selection of Variables

The observations in a clinical study involve two types of variables: outcome variables and influencing variables.

Outcome Variables   These variables should define and answer the research question and should have direct impact on the claims for the device.

- Also known as response, endpoints, or dependent variables
- Should be directly observable, objectively determined measures, and subject to minimal bias and error
- Should be directly related to biological effects

Influencing Variables   Any aspect of the study that can affect the outcome variables, or can affect the relationship between treatment and outcome, is an influencing variable.

- Also known as baseline variables, prognostic factors, confounding factors, or independent variables
- Are likely to affect the outcome, so extreme care should be taken to identify influencing variables. By taking known or suspected

variables into consideration, the sponsor minimizes the chance that conclusions drawn at the end of the study are spurious.

Study Population

The study population should be a representative subset of the population targeted for the application of the medical device. The study population should be defined before the start of the trial by the development of rigorous, unambiguous inclusion/exclusion criteria.

The advantage of using a restrictive population is that it allows for a smaller sample size in the clinical trial. The disadvantage is that it may limit the approval to a narrow subset of the general population as defined by the criteria.

Control Population

The preferred control group is an active control where patients are treated with a commercially available therapy. Less attractive is a placebo control (i.e., sham therapy), which usually raises ethical and enrollment issues. The least attractive control group is a historical control based on objective performance criteria (OPC).

Examples of the Different Control Groups   The control group in a clinical study could be an active parallel control groups, such as a placebo, or a current standard therapy for the selected condition. A concurrent control group could also be comprised of patients who refused to participate in the study and instead receive the alternative standard therapy. A historical control group consists of patients who share the disease symptoms with those in the active test group, but data from the historic control group were gathered from the medical literature in accordance to predetermined objective criteria. The following is a detailed discussion of these different control groups:

1. *Concurrent controls* are subjects who are assigned an alternative intervention, including no intervention or a placebo intervention, and are under the direct care of the clinical study investigator. Any concurrent control can be a treatment control if it is assigned another intervention. If a placebo or sham is assigned, then it becomes a placebo or sham control. If the controls do not receive any intervention, then they are called a "no treatment" control treatment. In a passive concurrent control design, subjects receive an alternative intervention,

including no intervention, but are not under the direct care of the study investigator.

2. *Self-controls or crossover controls* are subjects who are assigned one intervention (the order of treatment presentation should be specified in advance) for a prescribed period of time and then, following a washout period, receive the alternate intervention.

A washout period refers to a period of time in between the end of one experimental condition and the beginning of the next condition. The period of time between the two interventions should be based on current knowledge of how the device may affect any anatomical or physiological processes, so that it may be demonstrated that no residual effects of the first treatment remain that may confound the results obtained from the next scheduled treatment. It should be noted that there will still be instances where a subject may serve as his/her own control even if a crossover design is not necessary or appropriate. For example, a crossover design would not be necessary when it can be clearly demonstrated that current clinical consensus has determined that there are no residual effects of a device beyond the immediate treatment of the patient.

3. *An historical control* is a nonconcurrent group of subjects with the same disease or condition that have received an intervention (including no intervention) but are separated by time and usually place, from the population under the current study. Concurrent controls and, where applicable, self-controls allow the largest degree of opportunity for comparability.

Passive concurrent controls can provide comparability only if the selection criteria are the same, the study variables are measured in precisely the same way as those in the study sample, and assuming there are no hidden biases.

The use of historical controls is the most difficult way to ensure comparability with the study population, especially if the separation in time or place is large. The practice of medicine and nutrition is dynamic—hygiene and other factors change as well. Subtle differences (secular trends) in patient identification, concurrent therapies, or other factors can lead to differences in outcomes from a standard therapy or diagnostic algorithm. Such differences in patient selection, therapy, or other factors may not be easily or adequately documented. These differences in outcome may be mistakenly attributed to a new intervention when compared to a historical control observed at a significantly different time and/or place.

In addition it is often difficult or impossible to ascertain whether the measurement of critical study variables was sufficiently similar to those used in the current trial to allow comparison. It should not be assumed that the measurement methods are equivalent. For these reasons historical controls will usually require much more work to validate comparability with the study population than would concurrent controls.

If the sponsor and FDA agree to use a historic control for a particular clinical study, this historic control should be validated or adjusted in accordance with newly published research regarding this historic control group during the duration of the study. To explain this point further, the time difference between the approval of the IDE study and the submission of the PMA should be considered, where several new articles could be published to validate or dispute the historic control choice. Therefore the sponsor should always update the assumptions of the historic control based on this new published research.

Methods of Assigning Intervention

A method of assigning treatments or interventions to patients must minimize the potential for selection bias to enter the study. The preferred method for protecting the trial against selection bias is randomization. Generally, randomization methods utilize random number tables, computer-generated programs, and so forth. Specific methods of randomization with examples are discussed in textbooks[45-47] on clinical trials and medical statistics. The method of randomization used in a trial should be specified.

Specific Trial Designs[48,49]

There are numerous trial designs available to the sponsor. The choice of a particular design depends on many factors, including the hypotheses to be tested, number and impact of baseline characteristics on the outcome variable(s), number of study sites, and number of therapeutic or diagnostic categories to be measured.

The simplest and most common trial design is the *parallel design*. In this design a patient series from the study population has its baseline characteristics determined, is assigned one of two or more interventions, receives the assigned intervention, and is monitored at specified times after the intervention to determine outcome. If balance is achieved in the prognostic factors and follow-up is thorough, then the analysis and interpretation from a parallel design should be straightforward.

The crossover design[50] is a modification of the parallel design with the patient used as his/her own control. In this design each patient is assigned an order (presumably random) in which two or more interventions are to be given, followed by a period between interventions (or specimen collections) for a washout of any carryover effect from the previous intervention. These assignments should be made by randomization to protect against hidden or unknown biases. The conduct of a crossover design is somewhat more complicated than parallel designs and requires closer monitoring.

Analyses for crossover designs are also more complicated because the patient's response to any particular intervention is usually correlated with the response to another intervention. This is because more than one intervention is applied to the same patient and the response is likely to be influenced heavily by that patient's individual characteristics. However, patient-to-patient variability is controlled by employing a crossover design.

A third design that is applicable in medical device clinical trials is *the factorial design*. In a simple version of a factorial design, patients in the study population are assigned to one of four groups: one of two interventions under study, a control intervention, or both interventions. Such a trial may be used if a medical device was being tested against an alternate therapy, say a drug, and the research question is to determine if either intervention acting alone was effective, or if in combination they "interacted" to produce a stronger beneficial or detrimental effect.

The negative aspect of this design is that it is more complicated to conduct and the sponsor must ensure that investigators are adhering to the study protocol. A factorial design may require a larger sample size, but since this type of design is essentially two clinical trials in one, it offers an efficiency that should not be overlooked.

Other aspects of experimental design, such as *blocking* or *stratification*, may further complicate the evaluation. The design chosen for a particular study must be the one that is most applicable to the sponsor's objectives. These objectives may appropriately result in complicated studies that need to be developed, monitored, and evaluated carefully. Sometimes less complicated designs can be used by limiting the scope of the trial. Such a move, however, should be very carefully considered because it will nearly always result in a restriction on the claims for the device.

Masking or Blinding

Three of the more serious biases that may occur in a clinical trial are *investigator bias*, *evaluator bias*, and *placebo or sham effect*. An investigator bias occurs when the investigator either consciously or subconsciously favors one group at the expense of others. Evaluator bias can be a type of investigator bias in which the evaluator intentionally or unintentionally shades the measurements to favor one intervention over another. Studies that have subjective or quality of life endpoints are particularly susceptible to this form of bias.

The *placebo or sham effect* is a bias that occurs when a patient is exposed to an inactive therapy mode but believes that he/she is being treated with an intervention and subsequently shows or reports improvement.

The evolution of medical device evaluation has demonstrated that it is often difficult or impossible to mask the patient or investigator because a placebo or convincing sham treatment may not be feasible. In such cases extra care must be exercised by the study staff to ensure that these biases are minimized by the evaluator being blinded to the assignment of patients to a particular intervention or control group.

Study Site and Investigator

Pooling of data across study sites and investigators is almost always necessary in order to attain the required sample size. Therefore it is important to carefully select qualified sites and experienced investigators in the study. For more details on pooling of data across study sites, see Chapter 6, "Final Clinical Study Report."

Sample Size and Statistical Power

This topic is discussed in Chapter 5, "Statistical Analysis Plan (SAP) and Biostatistics in Clinical Research," under the section entitled "Example of Study Hypothesis."

CLINICAL TRIALS' DESIGN ISSUES AND DATA ANALYSIS ISSUES

Examination of Data across Study Centers

This topic is discussed in Chapter 6, "Final Clinical Study Report," under section entitled "Examination of Data Across Study Sites."

Repeated Measurements[51]

In a single-arm study where the hypothesis is to compare pretreatment and posttreatment effect or to evaluate the effect of the device over follow-up periods, repeated measurements are performed. For example, in studying the effect of renal stents in improving kidney function, serum creatinine is repeatedly measured at baseline, postprocedures, and at several follow-up visits to demonstrate the effect of this therapy on kidney function.

Subgroup Analysis

This topic is also discussed in greater detail in Chapter 6, "Final Clinical Study Report." Planned subgroup analysis can test for significant effects within subgroups. When the device effect is only significant for a certain subgroup, then inferences should be adjusted for multiple comparisons. Another advantage of this type of analysis is the selection of the population which will benefit most from the device in the subsequent trial.

Design Superiority and Noninferiority Compared

Superiority design shows that new treatment is better than the control or standard treatment. Efficacy trials are generally designed to answer the primary question of whether the new (experimental) intervention is superior in some way to the standard (control) intervention. The aim in such superiority trials is to rule out equality between the interventions by rejecting the null hypothesis that there is no difference between the two treatments. A common mistake is when a superiority trial fails to reject the null is to conclude that the two interventions being compared are equivalent when lack of superiority is evident. However, although lack of proof of superiority may be consistent with equivalence, it is not proof that equivalence is present.

The goal in an equivalence trial is to rule out differences of clinical importance in the primary outcome between the two treatments. The null hypothesis (in contrast with that in a superiority trial) is stated as a minimum difference that is acceptable and would render the two treatments interchangeable. The execution of an equivalence trial becomes an ambitious exercise because, by necessity, *it requires a much larger sample size than a superiority trial* and is less feasible to conduct.

Noninferiority Noninferiority trials show that the new treatment is not worse than the standard by more than a defined margin. An equivalence trial is appropriate when it is desired to demonstrate equivalence between two treatments, regimens, or interventions (methods) or noninferiority of a new one compared to a standard treatment. The conduct of an equivalence trial requires different techniques during design and analysis compared to a superiority trial.

Noninferiority Trial

- Uses active (positive) controls
- Addresses whether new (easier or cheaper) treatment is as good as the current treatment
- Must specify margin of "equivalence" or noninferiority
- Shows that the difference between the treatments is less than something with specified probability, since equivalency cannot be proved statistically
- Depends on historical evidence of sensitivity to treatment

A small sample size, leading to low power and subsequently lack of significant difference, does not imply "equivalence." Two examples will be used to illustrate the difference between superiority and noninferiority clinical trial. The first example includes the use of an ACE inhibitor for the treatment of high-risk MI patients. The second example describes the use of drug eluting stents in coronary artery disease patients.

The "Optimal" Trials:*[52]** ***Optimal Trial in Myocardial Infarction with the Angiotensin II Antagonist Losartan   The rationale for this study was as follows:

- ACE inhibitors reduce mortality in high-risk post-MI patients.
- Selective Angiotensin II receptor antagonists are an alternative because they more completely block the tissue renin-angiotensin system (RAS).
- Better tolerability is the working hypothesis.
- Losartan (50 mg) is superior or noninferior to captopril (150 mg) in decreasing all-cause mortality in high-risk patients following AMI study design.
- Study was designed as double-blind, randomized, parallel, investigator initiated, no placebo control.
- Event-driven study outcome was all-cause death (937), 499 in the losartan group and 447 in the captopril arm.

- A total of 5477 patients, in the multicenter study, were spread over Denmark, Finland, Germany, Ireland, Norway, Sweden, and the United Kingdom.
- Captopril was the comparator.
- Captopril has well-documented benefits.
- Captopril 50 mg 3 times daily has indication for Chronic Heart Failure (CHF) worldwide.
- Captopril is widely used, and available as a generic drug.

Study Results   The Angiotensin II antagonist losartan failed to show benefit over the ACE inhibitor captopril in this trial. Captopril showed a more positive trend toward superiority. The primary endpoint, all cause mortality, indicated that a total of 937 deaths was reported: 447 in the captopril (16.2%) and 499 (18.2%) in the losartan arm, with a *p*-value of 0.069 and 95% CI of 1.13 (0.99–1.28). However, losartan showed significant better tolerability than captopril.

New Drug Eluting Stent (DES) Study Design Challenges[53]   The trial design of new DES faced several challenges:

- Bare metal stent (BMS) controlled trial—the use of BMS as the control group is no longer feasible because of availability of the DES in the market
- Active controlled trial—noninferiority approach
- Operator technique—more aggressive to treat more complex lesions, more direct stenting

Superiority over DES?
- Current stent technologies have reduced the incidence of remaining safety and efficacy rates to between 5% and 8%.
- Proof of superiority of attempts to further reduce these events will require at least 14,000 patient studies with long-term follow-up, which is hardly infeasible.

Safety Endpoint—MACE Definition   A major adverse coronary event is a composite endpoint of

1. Cardiac death
2. MI (non-Q-wave and Q-wave)
3. Target vessel revascularization (TVR)

Target lesion revascularization (TLR) and non-TLR was the endpoint used in DES trials. Although a small increase in the incidence of very late stent thrombosis (after 1 year) with DES vs. BMS was reported, no evidence of associated increased mortality or MI with DES vs. BMS was seen. Also the marked benefit of DES upon the need to repeat revascularization was reconfirmed. So the trade-off between DES and BMS is a rare malignant (stent thrombosis) observed in the DES compared with more frequent restenosis in the BMS.

USE OF HISTORIC CONTROLS AS THE CONTROL GROUP IN IDE STUDIES[54-57]

The selection of "historic control" instead of employing an active control group in medical devices pivotal clinical trials remains to be one of the challenging issues in designing clinical studies. Randomized clinical studies are considered the golden standard for designing clinical trials, however, the use of this design may be unnecessary, inappropriate, or even impossible under certain circumstances. For example, the use of randomized clinical studies is impossible if it raises serious ethical concerns because of risks associated with patients in the control group. Additionally the use of RCT may be unnecessary when the effect of the intervention is dramatic, the use of interventional therapy in life-threatening conditions where it could be dramatic reduction of mortality. Finally, the use of RCT may be inappropriate to observe effects over long follow-up periods, such as assessments of orthopedic implants that require long-term follow-up periods. It should be noted that the use of historic controls is considered by the FDA and the scientific community as the least preferred type of control, and it shouldn't be used unless there is good evidence to support the design. The main reason for not using the historic control design in clinical studies is the elimination of bias in subject selection and other biases, as will be discussed below. Scientific and regulatory challenges facing the use of the historic control can be summarized as follows:

- The inherent variability in the historic control data may lead to erroneous conclusions regarding the effectiveness of the experimental treatment.
- Issues associated with selection of the historic control:
  - Historic control data should be presented in a reliable, accessible database.

- The sponsor should explain thoroughly the scientific arguments supporting proposed historic control design. For example, if the sponsor elects to use an objective criteria performance goal approach, the specific literature, and rationale justifying this approach should be explained in details.
- The sponsor should provide scientific evidence to match the subject's characteristics of the investigational treatment arm and the historic control arm.
- It should be clarified whether the historic control is selected from one or multiple studies?
- It should be clarified whether or not the database of selected historic control include detailed individual patient information?
- It is important to indicate whether or not the selected historic control is validated as new studies are published?

In this section important issues will be discussed: When might it be appropriate to use this type of noncontrol comparison in medical device pivotal studies? When objective performance criteria (OPC) can be used? What are the advantages and disadvantages for using OPC for historic controls? Additionally this section will include a discussion of recent FDA PMA studies as examples for accepting or rejecting the utilization of historic controls.

Definition of the Historic Control

The term "historic control" implies that individuals treated in the past are used as a comparison group for data analyzed of a study that had no control group. The definition implies the following:

- Current therapy and patients are studied against others in previous trials.
- The study is not randomized to current conditions.
- The historic control may be too far removed in time.

Objective Performance Criteria (OPC)

Objective performance criteria (OPC) is defined as the criteria agreed upon by the FDA to set specific limits to the selected historic control. These criteria are based on broad sets of data from historical databases (e.g., literature or registries) that are generally recognized as acceptable values. These criteria may be used for surrogate or clinical endpoints in demonstrating the safety or effectiveness of a device.

Advantages of OPCs   The advantages of predetermining OPC for the selected historic control are mainly viewed as the advantages of using historic controls, as this will lead to smaller sample size, will provide standard value for all sponsors, will ultimately save time and money, and will make the study easier to execute.

Disadvantages of OPCs   The disadvantages associated with OPCs are those problems associated with historic control, such as single-arm trials, selection bias, controls regarding data validity and analysis, and smaller sample size studies ($N = 100$ or 150). Additionally sometimes it is very difficult to validate the data of the historic controls.

When OPCs Might Be Used?   Historic controls can be used in certain circumstances if the following information is available:

- A great deal is known about the natural history of the disease or condition.
- Underlying patient population is well described and relatively stable.
- Extensive clinical history and experience with this device are available.
- Standard of care is stable and well known.
- No significant new questions of safety or effectiveness arise.
- Consensus exists among FDA, industry, clinical, and academic and patient communities.
- A significantly positive treatment effect can be expected.

What Should the Agreement with the FDA Contain?[53–56]
- Clear definitions of all appropriate terms
- Provisions for periodic updating of OPC
- Specific guidance on methodology to derive an OPC
- Unambiguous policy regarding failure to meet OPC

How to Determine OPC?
- Past, similar, approved devices
- Point estimate or that study's OPC

Examples of Clinical Studies with Historic Controls

In this section two examples of clinical studies that used historic control as the control group will be discussed in detail. The first study is the LACI clinical trial where the FDA Panel voted (9–1) for not approval decision. The Panel cited concerns that the choice of a control group for the study and data might be insufficient to support the effectiveness of the device. The second study is the ARCHeR trial in which the FDA approved the carotid stenting device.

LACI Clinical Study[58]   LACI (laser angioplasty for critical limb ischemia) clinical trial is an IDE study that was designed as a single-arm registry, prospective, and multicenter (US and international sites) study. The design of the study was as follow:

- Patient population: patients with critical limb ischemia (CLI)
  - Rutherford category 4–6
  - Poor surgical candidates
- Treatment: ELA of SFA, popliteal and/or infrapopliteal arteries, with adjunctive PTA and optional stenting
- Primary safety endpoint: any death occurrence in 6 months
- Primary effectiveness endpoint: percentage of alive patients without major amputations at 6 months
- Included catheters:
  - 2.2- to 2.5-mm spectranetics peripheral laser catheters
  - Any spectranetics coronary laser catheter
- Study patients considered poor surgical candidates because of:
  - Poor or absent vessel for outflow anastamosis
  - Absence of venous conduit
  - Significant comorbidity
- Enrollment period: April 2001 to April 2002
- Enrollment: 145 patients, 155 limbs at 14 sites in and outside the United States

Study Devices
- Excimer laser atherectomy (ELA)
- XeCl excimer laser, 308 nm, pulsed at 40 pulses/second maximum
- A fiber optic catheter first approved by FDA in 1993 for use in coronary arteries

Selection of the Control Group   The selected control group was selected based on the following criteria:

- Standard of care
- Indicated for LACI patients

Candidate Control Therapies
- Medication (conservative therapy)
- Primary amputation
- PTA + optional stents
- Bypass surgery

Randomization Not Considered   Randomization to an appropriate control group could not be achieved for the following reasons:

- No one therapy of the options listed above is appropriate, ethical, and standard of care for this population
- Randomization would be unworkable

Justification for Selection of Historic Control

Why Not Randomize versus Medications?   Randomizing against a treatment plan that promises 37% major amputation at 6 months has ethical issues. In the absence of LACI, patients at high risk of surgical mortality would receive medication and bed rest. The TransAtlantic Iner-Societal Consensus (TASC)[59] recommends only prostanoids, and then only when revascularization has failed or is impossible.

Why Not Randomize versus Amputation?   Randomizing against a treatment plan that promises 100% major amputation with a high death rate, both perioperative and long term, has ethical issues. It might be proposed that patients who are not at a high risk of surgical mortality may better benefit from primary amputation. Patients receiving primary amputation are at risk for perioperative mortality, long hospital stay, and high incidence of secondary amputation.

Why Not Randomize versus Bypass?   Bypass surgery is the "gold standard" for treatment of CLI. However, LACI patients were poor surgical candidates (bypass was not a treatment option). LACI patients who were poor surgical candidates presented one of the following conditions:

- High risk of surgical mortality
- Lack of distal anastomosis site
- Lack of venous conduit for bypass

Why Not Randomize versus PTA?   PTA is not recommended for all disease patterns in CLI (TASC recommendations),[55] and evidence that PTA can be successful in CLI/poor surgical candidates is lacking. This is a question of ethics in the control group. According to TASC recommendations, PTA was recommended for the vast majority of patients enrolled in this trial.

Best-Case Historical Control   The following points should be considered when selecting the historic control for this study:

- Exact match in patient characteristics
- Huge enrollment
- Full statistics, excellent follow-up
- Treatment plan defines "standard" (in this case, a mixed set of modalities that uses best-case therapy for each patient)
- Conforms to TASC definitions

The Historical Control "ICAI Study"[60]   The historic control for the LACI registry was selected from another randomized drug trial treating CLI in 1560 patients:

- Italian multicenter randomized study of Prostaglandin E1 in CLI patients, with 771 in the alprostadil group and 789 in the control group
- Control group received variety of therapies (bypass, endarterectomy, medication, and a few PTAs); *Ann Intern Med* 1999;130: 412–21
- Conforms to TASC definitions and GCP

ICAI Study: Differences   ICAI differs from LACI slightly:

- ICAI enrolled CLI patients regardless of candidacy for surgery (35% of ICAI patients received surgery as their primary treatment option)
- LACI enrolled only poor surgical candidates

TASC Consensus   TASC document recommends PTA for CLI only in simple lesions:

• Type A: single stenoses <1 cm

TASC does not recommend PTA in:

• Type B: multiple short stenoses
• Type C: long stenoses; short occlusions
• Type D: occlusions >2 cm; diffuse disease
• surgery is recommended for type D

TASC Types in LACI   Data were insufficient in 2/155 cases.

TASC Lesion Type	LACI Legs $n = 155$
A: short stenoses	3 (2%)
B: multiple short lesions	13 (8%)
C: complex patterns	44 (28%)
D: long diffuse disease	93 (60%)

Results of the LACI Phase 2 Registry   Table 8.1 shows the significant percentage differences in baseline risk factors regarding male gender, current smoking, prior MI, prior stroke, diabetes mellitus, hypertension, dyslipidemia, and obesity for the LACI arm group and the selected historic control.

Table 8.2 shows that data for certain lesion characteristics such as reasons for poor surgical candidacy are not available for the historic control group.

TABLE 8.1   Patients Baseline Characteristics

	LACI	Control	p-Value
Mean age, years	72 ± 10	72 ± 10	ns
Men	53%	72%	*
Risk factors			
Smoking current	14%	25%	*
Prior MI	23%	15%	*
Prior stroke	21%	12%	*
Diabetes mellitus	66%	39%	*
Hypertension	83%	49%	*
Dyslipidemia	56%	16%	*
Obesity	35%	7%	*

Note: *indicates significant difference.

TABLE 8.2 Lesion Characteristics

	LACI	Control	p-Value
Rutherford category 4, 5, or 6	27%	30%	ns
	72%	70%	ns
Reasons for poor surgical candidacy			
Absence of venous graft	32%		
Poor/no distal vessel	68%		
High surgical risk	46%	11%	*
Only one reason	61%		
Any two reasons	33%		
All three reasons	6%		

Note: *indicates significant difference.

Planned Criteria Poor surgical candidates presented:

- $\geq$ASA Class 4
- Absence of SAV for conduit
- Extensive pathology

Actual Enrollment
- Only 46% met ASA criteria.
- Only 32% did not have SAV.
- Lesions: 41% SFA, 27% popliteal/tibio-peroneal, with mean of 2.7 lesions/limb, and mean length of 6 ± 7 cm
- Lesions were amenable to PTA?

Study Design
- The sponsor's objective was to show that the results in the treatment group were at least as good as for the control group—an equivalence design.
- FDA agreed to accept the equivalence design based on the assumption that the control patients would be less sick than the LACI registry patients.

The effectiveness primary endpoint was met as "percentage of alive patients without amputation at 6 months."

Equivalence Hypothesis
- Hypothesis: Equivalence to historical nonintervention control
- Sponsor: conservative comparison because LACI patients will be more comorbid and at greater risk for poor outcome

The outcome of the LACI study is shown in Tables 8.3 and 8.4.

TABLE 8.3   LACI Study Outcomes

Variable	LACI	ICAI
Patients enrolled	145	789
Censored/withdrawn	—	[116]
Patients for analysis	145	673
Lost to follow-up	11 (7.6%)	7 (1.0.%)
Patients not lost to follow-up	134	666
Deaths	15 (11.2%)	96 (14.4%)
Alive with amputation at 6 months	9 (7.6%)	76 (13.3%)
Limb salvage at 6 months	110 (75.9%)	494 (73.4%)
Persisting CLI	43 (29.7%)	211 (31.4%)
Serious AEs	58 (40.0%)	239 (35.5%)
Re-interventions	24 (17.9%)	34 (5.1%)

TABLE 8.4   The Primary Effectiveness Endpoint

LACI	Control
75.9% (110/145)	73.4% (494/673)

Note: 95% CI (−5.3%, 10.2%).

- Trial outcome showed that:
  - Only patient age predicted mortality and need for amputation (the same in LACI and ICAI studies)
  - Difficult to determine if one group was more sick than the other, given the differences in risk factors

Limitations to the Analysis of the Primary Endpoint   Nonrandomized study's visible differences were as follows:

- LACI and control patients were not comparable, mainly due to differences in rest pain, previous minor amputations, and previous major amputations
- Country and hospital factors were not comparable.

Historic control raw data at the patient level were not available:

- Visible differences could not be accounted for.
- Formal sensitivity analysis for hidden biases could not be carried out.

FDA Panel Discussion   Despite the fact that the LACI study met the primary endpoints of equivalence in 6-month limb salvage and death rates, the FDA and panel members were concerned that there is not enough evidence to justify from the data the assumption that the patients in the LACI registry would be more comorbid and at greater risk for poor outcome, compared to the control group. The major weaknesses of the selected control were that the selection was based on one study and access to detailed patients' data was not available, and so raised concern about the comparability of the patients in the control group and active test group.

ACCULINK™ Carotid Stent System and RX ACCULINK™ Carotid Stent System

Study Design[61]   The ACCULINK for revascularization of carotids in high-risk patients (ARCHeR) clinical trials were a series of prospective, nonrandomized, multicenter, single-arm clinical trials. These trials were performed to demonstrate the safety and efficacy of the ACCULINK™ and RX ACCULINK™ carotid stent systems with embolic protection to treat high-risk, surgical and nonsurgical symptomatic ($\geq 50\%$ stenosis) and asymptomatic ($\geq 80\%$ stenosis) subjects with disease in the internal carotid artery. A total of 581 patients were enrolled at 45 clinical sites in the United States and five sites outside of the United States. The design of the trial was as follows:

ARCHeR 1 evaluated the over-the-wire (OTW) ACCULINK™ carotid stent system and included 158 registry patients. The primary objective of the study was to determine if the occurrence rate of the composite primary endpoint of stroke, death, and myocardial infarction (MI) at 30 days and ipsilateral stroke at one year for carotid stenting is not inferior to the occurrence rate of carotid endarterectomy (CEA) in the population under evaluation.

ARCHeR 2 evaluated the OTW ACCULINK™ carotid stent system and OTW ACCUNET™ embolic protection system and included 278 registry patients. The primary objective of the study was the same as for ARCHeR 1. The second primary endpoint for this study was ACCUNET™ device success.

ARCHeR 3 evaluated the rapid exchange (RX) ACCULINK™ carotid stent system and RX ACCUNET™ embolic protection system and included 145 patients. The primary objective of the study was to establish equivalence (noninferiority) to the ARCHeR 2 results with respect to 30-day death, stroke, and MI as a means of establishing equivalency between the OTW and RX devices.

The Historic Control Assumptions The historic control for this trial was based on OPC that was derived from multiple clinical studies, including the following land mark studies:

- NASCET[62], North American Symptomatic Carotid Endarterectomy Trial. Methods, patient characteristics, and progress. *Stroke* 1991;22(6):711–20.
- North American Symptomatic Carotid Endarterectomy Trial[63]: Barnett HJ, Taylor DW, Eliasziw M, Fox AJ, Ferguson GG, Haynes RB, Rankin RN, Claggett GP, Hachinski VC, Sackett DL, Thorpe KE, Meldrum HE. Benefit of carotid endarterectomy in patients with symptomatic moderate or severe stenosis. North American Symptomatic Carotid Endarterectomy Trial Collaborators. *N Engl J Med* 1998;339(20):1415–25.
- ACAS[64], Endarterectomy for Asymptomatic Carotid Artery Stenosis. Executive Committee for the Asymptomatic Carotid Atherosclerosis Study. *JAMA* 1995;273(18):1421–8.

The OPC proposed for this studies continued to be validated by newly published studies, particularly the SAPPHIRE trial, which was presented to the FDA few months before the ACCULINK PMA submission.

The study hypothesis of the ARCHeR 1 and ARCHeR 2 trials was to show equivalence (noninferiority) between carotid stenting and an historical control, based on the standard of care. The historical control was established based on a review of the current literature on carotid endarterectomy and medical therapy. From this review the rate of 30-day death, stroke, MI and ipsilateral stroke at 31 to 365 days was estimated at 15% for patients with medical comorbidities and estimated at 11% for patients with anatomy unfavorable for CEA. A weighted historical control (WHC) was calculated based on the proportion of each of these patient groups enrolled in the study.

$$WHC = pc * 15\% + pa * 11\%,$$

where pc = the proportion of patients with medical comorbidities and pa = the proportion of patients with unfavorable anatomy. Using this equation, the *WHC* rate at one year was calculated for both ARCHeR 1 and ARCHeR 2 to be 14.5%. The ARCHeR 3 trial was designed to demonstrate equivalence (noninferiority) of the safety and performance of the rapid exchange RX ACCULINK™ and RX ACCUNET™ systems to results observed in the ARCHeR 2 trial for the OTW ACCULINK™ and ACCUNET™ systems based on 30-day results.

The primary objectives of the ARCHeR 1 and ARCHeR 2 trials were met. The upper confidence limits for primary endpoint rates fell below the 14.5% *WHC* for both studies, demonstrating that carotid stenting is noninferior to carotid endarterectomy in the studied high-risk population.

The primary objective of the ARCHeR 3 study, that the 30-day primary endpoint for the ARCHeR 3 study was noninferior to that of the ARCHeR 2 study, was met. The upper bound of the 95% confidence interval of the difference between ARCHeR 3 and ARCHeR 2 is 4.75%, which is less than the delta of 8% ($p = 0.005$). Thus results from ARCHeR 3 are determined to be noninferior to those of ARCHeR 2, and the RX and OTW devices are determined to yield similar clinical results.

Advantage of the Choice of the Historic Control in the ARCHeR Trial

1. The historic control was based on numerous clinical studies with similar patient criteria to those enrolled in the trial.
2. The historical control data were validated in accordance with the newly published research, from the time of the IDE submission until the PMA submission (5 years), and this validation supported the originally proposed *WHC*.
3. The historic control was supported by other randomized clinical studies (the SAPPHIRE study) that were submitted and recommended for approval by the FDA panel just before the submission of the ACCULINK PMA.

CDRH Decision   FDA issued an approval order in August 2004. The RX and OTW ACCULINK carotid stent systems were granted expedited review status in April 2004 because these devices could offer a viable alternative to the current standard of care for patients with carotid artery disease. Because these devices may represent a reduced risk compared to existing technology, the FDA granted expedited review to the ACCULINK™ carotid stent system and RX ACCULINK™ carotid stent system.

SUMMARY OF RECOMMENDATIONS WHEN USING HISTORIC CONTROLS

The following recommendations are set forward for study sponsors when they are considering the use of historic control in a clinical trial:

1. Historic control is mainly selected if randomization to the control group raises ethical concerns because of risks associated with patients in the control group.
   a. The trials designed to treat life-threatening conditions.
   b. The benefit of the investigational device could be dramatic.
   c. The investigational therapy could have a dramatic effect in reducing mortality.
2. Historic control data should be present in a reliable database where access is available to prevent lack of information in comparison parameters.
3. When possible the historic control should be selected from multiple studies or multiple databases.
4. It is important to validate the historic control data as new studies are published.
5. Patients' baseline characteristics in the proposed study and those of the historic control group should be comparable.
6. If the historic control is based on international studies, then country and hospital factors should be considered.
7. Historic controls can be used in certain circumstances if the following information is available:
   a. Much is known about the natural history of the disease or condition.
   b. Underlying patient population is well described and relatively stable.
   c. Extensive clinical history and experience with this device exists.
   d. Standard of care is stable and well known.
   e. No significant new questions of safety or effectiveness arise.
   f. Consensus exists among FDA, industry, clinical, academic, and patient communities.
   g. Significantly positive treatment effect can be expected.

8. Study's sponsor should agree with the FDA regarding the OPC for the historic control:
   a. Clear definitions of all appropriate terms
   b. Provisions for periodic updating of OPC
   c. Specific guidance on methodology to derive an OPC
   d. Unambiguous policy regarding failure to meet OPC

9

INVESTIGATOR-INITIATED CLINICAL RESEARCH

Investigator-initiated clinical studies are becoming more common, particularly in academic institutions funded by federal sources or private industry. To understand this type of research, it is important to answer the following key questions: Who are the parties? What are their roles? What is the purpose of the research?

Unlike clinical studies sponsored by biopharmaceutical or medical device companies, the sponsor of investigator-initiated research is usually an academic institution or private group of investigators. The

Design, Execution, and Management of Medical Device Clinical Trials,
by Salah Abdel-aleem
Copyright © 2009 John Wiley & Sons, Inc.

sponsor of the study is usually responsible for the financial support, protocol development, product provision, conduct, and management of the study.

Investigator-initiated clinical research is undertaken to achieve the following objectives:

- Improve science/data
- Optimize patient benefit
- Support a new use/indication of a drug or medical device
- Support product strategy

These studies can also be achieved through the following submission mechanisms:

- Traditional IND/IDE
- Non–IND/IDE drug or device studies
- Nondrug or device studies

DEFINITION AND EXAMPLES OF INVESTIGATOR-INITIATED CLINICAL RESEARCH

The Investigator is defined as an individual (not a corporation) who both initiates (plans and designs) and conducts an investigation, and under whose immediate direction the investigational therapy is administered or dispensed. In other words, the investigator plans, designs, conducts, monitors, manages the data; prepares reports; and oversees all regulatory and ethical matters. The investigator is responsible for developing the clinical protocol, study budget, study resources (project management, regulatory guidance, data management, facilities and clinical labs, obtaining the study product, etc.). The investigator is also responsible for getting approval from regulatory and funding agents (e.g., IRB, FDA, and NIH). Investigator-initiated clinical studies are usually conducted for an unapproved FDA product, but the investigation could be of an already approved FDA product to expand its use to a new indication or a new patient population.

Requirements of the Investigator-Initiated Clinical Research

Protocol   The protocol is left to the investigator to author. The funding source for the investigator-initiated clinical trials may be a for-profit entity, a nonprofit foundation, or a charitable organization.

Resources
- Data management and biostatistical support
- Study monitoring
- Regulatory consultants
- Collaboration with a drug or medical device company to provide investigational products
- Legal assistance

Publication and Mandatory Registration Requirements The FDA Amendments Act, mandates registration of Phases II to IV clinical trials of drugs and biologics, and devices. In addition the International Committee of Medical Journal Editors (ICMJE) requires all new clinical research studies to be entered in a public registry at or before the onset of subject enrollment.

Intellectual Property Rights for Investigator Intellectual property rights issues should be carefully considered when planning an investigator-initiated clinical research:

- Know whether the university, or place of work of the investigator, retains all rights to inventions developed under the study.
- If the funding source for the clinical trial is a for-profit entity, the entity will be granted the first right to negotiate for a license to commercialize the invention.
- If the funding source is a nonprofit entity, the nonprofit entity will be granted certain noncommercial rights to the invention.

Subject Injury for Investigator
- Except for injury attributable to the manufacture of the study investigational product, the university or place of work of the investigator assumes responsibility for any injury directly resulting from the subject participation in the investigator-initiated trial.
- The university or place of work of the investigator will provide medical treatment for any such injuries.
- It is unacceptable to require billing of third-party insurance companies in lieu of recovery of such costs.

Potential Risk Perspective

The following risks are associated with the industry, investigator, or institution participating in this type of research:

Industry

- Ineffective use of resources (financial and personnel) in that they do not support the strategic plan
- Lack of up-front planning in that trial leads to potential nonvalidated data that cannot be utilized for publication or support of FDA submission
- Data results that oppose current data results or strategic plan
- Inappropriate budgets suggesting marketing influence
- Legal issues from noncompliance

Institution/Investigator

- Local sponsorship ambiguity
- Inadequate resources to act as sponsor
- Presentation/publication of data that might not have been validated
- Pivotal impact for research subject safety
- Legal issues from noncompliance to regulation
- Lack of indemnification of site from funding sources

DEVELOPMENT, CONDUCT, AND MANAGEMENT OF INVESTIGATOR-INITIATED CLINICAL RESEARCH

The development of investigator-initiated clinical research takes the following chronological steps:

- Project development
  - Letter of intent
  - Proposal
  - Timeline
  - Protocol development and data collection forms
  - Budget development
  - Funding
- Contract
- IRB review and approval
- Study conduct and monitoring
- Data review and analysis

What Is the Letter of Intent (LOI)?

- Statement of your research interest in a particular drug or device
- Your interest in conducting a clinical trial with the drug or device
- Type of human research participant population
- Anticipated time to conduct the trial
- Funding source
- Who will supply the drug or device

What Should Be in the LOI?

- Rationale for the proposed trial
- Design for the trial (dose, blinding, schedule, and comparison groups)
- Characteristics of the population
- Patient enrollment feasibility
- Any unique features of the proposed trial (who would benefit from the new information? patients? industry?)

Project Timeline

Development phase:

- Regulatory (IRB, FDA, NIH) and legal (contract)
- Project conduct phase
  - Recruitment
  - Trial conduct
  - Data collection
  - Data quality assurance
- Data review and analysis
- Publication

REGULATION OF INVESTIGATOR-INITIATED CLINICAL RESEARCH

Investigator-initiated clinical research should follow all the following regulations and guidelines:

- Federal regulation
- ICH guidelines
- State laws
- Institutional policy
- Contractual agreements
- The protocol
- Investigator SOPs

REQUIRED INFRASTRUCTURE FOR INVESTIGATOR-INITIATED CLINICAL RESEARCH

The following infrastructure is required for investigator initiated clinical research:

Conduct and Management of the Study

- Monitoring regulatory submissions
- Oversight of study conduct (e.g., qualification and education of staff)
- Oversight of data and research subject safety

Financial Budgets

Ensure that the projected budget is representative of full study costs.

- Personnel
- Procedures
- Supplies
- Facilities
- Recruitment
- Training
- Monitoring

Contract Financial Considerations

- A written budgetary agreement should be in place, specifying the type of the research services to be provided and the basis for payment for those services.

- Investigator compensation should be reasonable for services performed.
- Payment should not be tied to study outcome.
- The investigator team (or their families) should not have conflict of interest related to the product being studied.

CLINICAL RESEARCH SPONSORED BY NIH

The National Institute of Health (NIH) has created the Clinical Research Policy Analysis and Coordination (CRPAC) Program to harmonize, streamline, and optimize policies and requirements concerning the conduct and oversight of clinical research. The CRPAC Program was created to promote the efficiency and effectiveness of the clinical research enterprise, in part by facilitating compliance and oversight.

CRPAC staff work closely with other federal agencies including the Office for Human Research Protections, the Food and Drug Administration, the Department of Veterans Affairs, the Department of Defense, and other federal agencies that have adopted the federal policy for the protection of human subjects.

Some specific objectives of this program regarding policies in clinical research are as follows:

- Coordinating diverse adverse event reporting requirements
- Clarifying the respective roles and responsibilities of data safety and monitoring boards (DSMBs) and other review mechanisms
- Clarifying policy where variability in the application of the human subjects regulations exists
- Examining the characteristics and features of various models of IRB review and considering their advantages for forms of research activities
- Studying various approaches to providing informed consent and sharing best practices, and creating dialogue on promoting science, safety, and ethics through clinical trial design

10

ETHICAL CONDUCT FOR HUMAN RESEARCH

The principals for ethical conduct of human clinical research were derived from:

- Nuremberg Code, 1974
- Declaration of Helsinki, 1964
- Belmont Report, 1978

The principles of the ethical conduct for research involving humans are summarized as follows[65–67]:

- *Social and Clinical Value for Society and Patients*   Clinical trials should be designed to provide a significant value for society or for patients, both present and future, with a particular illness. The study should contribute to our scientific understanding of disease, its

Design, Execution, and Management of Medical Device Clinical Trials,
by Salah Abdel-aleem
Copyright © 2009 John Wiley & Sons, Inc.

diagnosis, and treatment. Human subjects may be subjected to risks associated with participating in the trial only if society will gain useful knowledge.

- *Scientific Validity of the Study*   The clinical study should follow valid scientific methods in order to achieve the research objectives in a scientific manner.
- *Fair Subject Selection*   This process ensures fair selection of study subjects who fit all of the study eligibility criteria and are enrolled in the study. The study design must ensure that neither privileged nor vulnerable subjects are allowed in the study.
- *Favorable Risk/Benefit Ratio*   Research risks may be trivial or serious, and they may cause transient discomfort or long-term changes. All efforts must be made to minimize the risks and inconvenience to research subjects, to maximize the potential benefits, and to determine that the potential benefits to individuals and society are proportionate to, or outweigh, the risks. In certain studies, such as feasibility studies, there are no direct benefits to participating subjects, but society at large and/or future patients will benefit.
- *Independent Review*   The independent review process of clinical studies can be done through the IRB, DSMB, or other granting agencies to minimize potential conflicts of interest and to make sure a study is ethically acceptable before it starts. These groups also monitor a study while it is ongoing.
- *Informed Consent*   One of the most important items in any clinical study is the subject consent for the participation in the trial. This is done through a process of informed consent in which individuals (1) are accurately informed of the purpose, methods, risks, benefits, and alternatives to the research; (2) understand this information and how it relates to their own clinical situation or interests; and (3) make a voluntary decision about whether to participate.
- *Respect for Potential and Enrolled Subjects*   Individuals should be treated with respect from the time they are screened for possible participation—even if they refuse enrollment in a study—throughout their participation and after their participation ends.

THE NUREMBERG CODE (1947)

The Nuremberg Code states certain basic principles that must be observed in order to satisfy moral, ethical, and legal concepts for the protection of patients. Three pivotal principles of the Nuremberg Code have laid down conditions for ethical research:

1. Obtain consent from the research subject
2. Conduct animal experiments first
3. Supervise the research

WORLD MEDICAL ASSOCIATION—DECLARATION OF HELSINKI (1964–PRESENT)

Key elements of the Declaration of Helsinki are summarized as follows:

1. Physicians' responsibility is to protect the life, health, privacy, and dignity of the human subject.
2. Research must follow accepted scientific guidelines.
3. Welfare of the environment and animals must be respected.
4. Protocol must be submitted to an ethical review committee:
   Ethical considerations must be explained.
   Prediction of risks, burdens, and benefits should be explained.
5. Research should only be conducted by scientifically qualified persons.
6. Each potential subject must be informed, made to understand, and be free to consent after the material facts of the study are explained.
7. Consent must be given without coercion:
   Legal guardians must provide consent for those that cannot.
   Minors must assent to the research.
8. Researchers must utilize scientific integrity in reporting findings.

NATIONAL COMMISSION FOR THE PROTECTION OF HUMAN SUBJECTS OF BIOMEDICAL AND BEHAVIORAL RESEARCH (1974)

Instituted by the 1974 *National Research Act*
   Required Institutional Review Boards (IRBs): 45 CFR 46 ("Title 45 of the Code of Federal Regulations: Chapter 46").

THE BELMONT REPORT (1978)

- Respect for persons (autonomy)
- Informed consent
- Beneficence/nonmalfeasance
- Assessment of potential risks and benefits
- Justice
- Fair selection of participants

SPECIAL ETHICAL CONCERNS IN CLINICAL RESEARCH ON USE OF PLACEBO

The fifth revision of the Declaration of Helsinki included a principle that stated, "The benefits, risks, burdens and effectiveness of a new method should be tested against the best current prophylactic, diagnostic and therapeutic method."

This seemed to preclude the use of a placebo in clinical research whenever standard treatment is available. Although this statement was subsequently clarified to not preclude all uses of placebos, it intensified the long-standing discussion of and concern *about placebo use* and the ethical review of clinical research between the welfare of individual subjects and the benefit to society. Some of these studies would have been considered to be unethical in most developed countries, but were justified on the basis of a different local standard of care. This raises the question of whether ethics requires that the practices in all parts of the world be identical.

Use of a placebo raises the dilemma of potential subject harm and the scientific validity of the study. The range of opinions regarding the use of a placebo in clinical research varies between two extreme positions:

1. The insistence on placebo-controlled trials, which consider that a placebo is the preferred comparator unless it exposes the subject to death or irreversible, severe damage, provided that the subject consents to participate and tolerate the risks and discomforts of the investigation.
2. The categorical objection to the use of a placebo, which maintains that whenever standard treatment exists, the use of a placebo is unethical. In such situations research treatments should be compared with standard treatments.

All parties agree that *the use of a placebo is unacceptable in life-threatening diseases* or in case of potential irreversible damage when there effective treatment exists, but the dilemma persists as to whether it is ethical to deprive subjects of standard treatment and expose them to a lesser degree to risk and discomfort.

Some bioethicists agree that if a placebo is required for scientific validity in a research study, this constitutes one ethical argument in favor, though not the full justification, of the use of the placebo. An appeal to the subject's autonomy is another justification for the use of a placebo.

This argument relies heavily on the disclosure of the risks of a placebo in the process of informed consent; however, some believe that this just transfers the ethical burden to the research subject. The ethical acceptability of disclosure as a justification for the use of a placebo depends on the subject's capacity to understand the implications of participating in a research study.

Federal regulations and international guidelines rely on independent ethical review to help ensure that research subjects are not exposed to unnecessary risks, including those presented by the use of a placebo.

GLOSSARY OF CLINICAL TRIAL AND STATISTICAL TERMS

Absolute risk difference   The difference in size of risk between two groups. For example, if one group has a 15% risk of contracting a particular disease, and the other has a 10% risk of getting the disease, the risk difference is five percentage points.

Adjusted analysis   An analysis that controls (adjusts) for baseline imbalances in important patient characteristics.

Adverse effect   An adverse event for which the causal relation between the drug/intervention and the event is at least a reasonable possibility. The term adverse effect applies to all interventions.

Adverse reaction   (adverse event) An unwanted effect caused by the administration of drugs. Onset may be sudden or develop over time.

Approved drugs   In the United States the FDA must approve drugs through a process that involves several steps, including preclinical laboratory and animal studies, investigational new drug (IND) application to start clinical trials for safety and efficacy, and filing of a new drug application (NDA) by the manufacturer of the drug. The drug is approved after the FDA approves the NDA.

Design, Execution, and Management of Medical Device Clinical Trials,
by Salah Abdel-aleem
Copyright © 2009 John Wiley & Sons, Inc.

Arm   Any of the treatment groups in a randomized trial. Most randomized trials have two "arms," but some have three "arms," or even more.

Attrition   The loss of participants during the course of a study (also called patients loss to follow-up). Participants that are lost during the study are often call dropouts.

Baseline
1. Information gathered at the beginning of a study from which variations found in the study are measured.
2. Initial time point in a clinical trial, just before a participant starts to receive the experimental treatment that is being tested.

Bias   When a point of view prevents impartial judgment on issues relating to the subject of that point of view. In clinical studies, bias is controlled by several methods such as blinding and randomization.

Categorical data   Data that are classified into two or more nonoverlapping categories. Race and type of drug (aspirin, paracetamol, etc.) are examples of categorical variables. If there is a natural order to the categories, for example, nonsmokers, ex-smokers, light smokers, and heavy smokers, the data are known as ordinal data. If there are only two categories, the data are dichotomous data.

Causal effect   An association between two characteristics that can be demonstrated to be due to cause and effect, such as a change in one causes the change in the other. Causality can be demonstrated by experimental studies such as controlled trials (e.g., that an experimental intervention causes a reduction in mortality). However, causality can often not be determined from an observational study.

Censored   A term used in studies whose outcome is the time to a particular event, to describe data from patients where the outcome is unknown. A patient might be known not to have had the event only up to a particular point in time, so "survival time" is censored at this point.

Chi-squared test   A statistical test based on comparison of a test statistic to a chi-squared distribution. Used in RevMan analyses to test the statistical significance of the heterogeneity statistic.

Clinical investigator   A medical researcher in charge of carrying out a clinical trial's protocol.

Clinical trial   A research study to answer specific questions about new therapies or new ways of using known treatments. Clinical trials are used to determine whether new drugs or treatments are both safe and effective. Carefully conducted clinical trials are the fastest and safest way to find treatments that work in people.

Clinically significant   A result (e.g., a treatment effect) that is large enough to be of practical importance to patients and health care providers. The hypothesis of clinical studies is usually based on clinical significant effect. This is not the same thing as statistically significant. Assessing clinical significance takes into account factors such as the size of a treatment effect, the severity of the condition being treated, the side effects of the treatment, and the cost.

Cohort   In epidemiology, a group of individuals with some characteristics in common.

Comorbidity   The presence of one or more diseases or conditions other than those of primary interest. In a study looking at treatment for one disease or condition, some individuals may have other diseases or conditions that could affect their outcomes (comorbidity may be a confounder).

Compassionate use   A method of providing experimental therapeutics prior to final FDA approval for use in humans. This procedure is used with very sick individuals who have no other treatment options. Often case-by-case approval must be obtained from the FDA for "compassionate use" of a drug or therapy.

Confidence interval (CI)   A measure of the uncertainty around the main finding of a statistical analysis. Estimates of unknown quantities, such as the odds ratio comparing an experimental intervention with a control, are usually presented as a point estimate and a 95% confidence interval. This means that if someone were to keep repeating a study in other samples from the same population, 95% of the confidence intervals from those studies would contain the true value of the unknown quantity. Alternatives to 95%, such as 90% and 99% confidence intervals, are sometimes used. Wider intervals indicate lower precision; narrow intervals, greater precision.

Confidence limits   The upper and lower boundaries of a confidence interval.

Confounder   A factor that is associated with both an intervention (or exposure) and the outcome of interest. For example, if people in the experimental group of a controlled trial are younger than those in the control group, it will be difficult to decide whether a lower risk of death in one group is due to the intervention or the difference in ages. Age is then said to be a confounder, or a confounding variable. Randomization is used to minimize imbalances in confounding variables between experimental and control groups. Confounding is a major concern in non-randomized studies.

Continuous data   Data with a potentially infinite number of possible values within a given range. Height, weight, and blood pressure are examples of continuous variables.

Cross-over trial   A type of clinical trial comparing two or more interventions in which the participants, upon completion of the course of one treatment, are switched to another. For example, for a comparison of treatments A and B, the participants are randomly allocated to receive them in either the order A, B or the order B, A. Cross-over trials are particularly appropriate for study of treatment options for relatively stable health problems. The time during which the first interventions is taken is known as the first period, with the second intervention being taken during the second period.

Confidentiality regarding trial participants   Refers to maintaining the confidentiality of trial participants including their personal identity and all personal medical information. The trial participants' consent to the use of records for data verification purposes should be obtained prior to the trial and assurance must be given that confidentiality will be maintained.

Contraindication   A specific circumstance when the use of certain treatments could be harmful. Sometimes this term is confused with an entirely different term, namely the use of the product with precaution.

Control group   The standard by which experimental observations are evaluated. In many clinical trials one group of patients will be given an experimental drug or treatment, while the control group is given either a standard treatment for the illness or a placebo.

Controlled trials   Control is a standard against which experimental observations may be evaluated. In clinical trials one group of participants is given an experimental drug, while another group (i.e., the control group) is given either a standard treatment for the disease or a placebo.

Cost-effectiveness analysis   An economic analysis that views effects in terms of overall health specific to the problem, and describes the costs for some additional health gain.

Data safety and monitoring board (DSMB)   An independent committee composed of community representatives and clinical research experts that review data while a clinical trial is in progress to ensure that participants are not exposed to undue risk. A DSMB may recommend that a trial be stopped if there are safety concerns or if the trial objectives have been achieved.

Dependent variable   The outcome or response that results from changes to an independent variable. In a clinical trial, the outcome (over which the investigator has no direct control) is the dependent variable, and the treatment arm is the independent variable.

Diagnostic trials   Refers to trials that are conducted to find better tests or procedures for diagnosing a particular disease or condition. Diagnostic trials usually include people who have signs or symptoms of the disease or condition being studied.

Distribution   The collection of values of a variable in the population or the sample, sometimes called an empirical distribution.

Dose-ranging study   A clinical trial in which two or more doses of an agent (e.g., a drug) are tested against each other to determine which dose works best and is least harmful.

Dose dependent   A response to a drug that may be related to the amount received (i.e., the dose). Sometimes trials are done to test the effects of different dosages of the same drug. This may be true for both benefits and harms.

Dose-dependent range   The relationship between the quantity of treatment given and its effect on outcome. In meta-analysis, dose–response relationships can be investigated using meta-regression.

Double-blind study   A clinical trial design in which neither the participating individuals nor the study staff knows which participants are receiving the experimental drug and which are receiving a placebo (or another therapy). Double-blind trials are thought to produce objective results, since the expectations of the doctor and the participant about the experimental drug do not affect the outcome.

Drug–drug interaction   A modification of the effect of a drug when administered with another drug. The effect may be an increase or a decrease in the action of either substance, or it may be an adverse effect that is not normally associated with either drug.

Effectiveness   The extent to which a specific intervention, when used under ordinary circumstances, does what it is intended to do. For example, if the device is intended for pain relief, it is expected that the device will actually relieve pain, with evidence demonstrating this effect.

Efficacy   The extent to which an intervention produces a beneficial result under ideal conditions. Clinical trials that assess efficacy are sometimes called explanatory trials. Efficacy of a drug or treatment could be defined as the maximum ability of a drug or treatment to produce a result regardless of dosage. A drug passes efficacy trials if it is effective at the dose tested and against the illness for which it is prescribed.

Eligibility criteria   Summary criteria for participants' selection; included are inclusion and exclusion criteria.

Empirical   Based on experimental data, not on a theory.

Endpoint   Overall outcome that the protocol is designed to evaluate.

Epidemiology   The branch of medical science that deals with the study of incidence and distribution and control of a disease in a population.

Experimental drug   A drug that is not FDA licensed for use in humans, or as a treatment for a particular condition.

Equipoise   A state of uncertainty where a person believes it is equally likely that either of two treatment options is better.

Equivalence trial   A trial designed to determine whether the response to two or more treatments differs by an amount that is clinically unimportant. This is usually demonstrated by showing that the true treatment difference is likely to lie between a lower and an upper equivalence level of clinically acceptable differences.

Food and Drug Administration (FDA)   The US Department of Health and Human Services agency responsible for ensuring the safety and effectiveness of all drugs, biologics, and medical devices, including those used in the diagnosis, treatment, and prevention of diseases.

Good clinical practice (GCP)   Basically the rules for the design, conduct, performance, monitoring, auditing, recording, analysis, and reporting of clinical trials. GCP provide assurance that data and results are based on sound scientific and ethical research. They are a broad set of requirements, standards, and recommendations that apply to thousands of highly specific tasks.

Historical control   A control person or group for whom data were collected earlier than for the group being studied. There is a large risk of bias in studies that use historical controls due to systematic differences between the comparison groups, due to changes over time in risks, prognosis, health care, and so forth.

Hypothesis   A supposition or assumption advanced as a basis for reasoning or argument, or as a guide to experimental investigation.

Inclusion/exclusion criteria   The medical or social standards determining whether a person may or may not be allowed to enter a clinical trial. These criteria are based on such factors as age, gender, the type and stage of a disease, previous treatment history, and other medical conditions.

Informed consent   The process of learning the key facts about a clinical trial before deciding whether to participate. It is also a continuing process throughout the study to provide information for participants. To help someone decide whether to participate, the doctors and nurses involved in the trial explain the details of the study.

Informed consent document   A document that describes the rights of the study participants, and includes details about the study, such as its purpose, duration, required procedures, and key contacts. Risks and potential benefits are explained in the informed consent document. The participant then decides whether to sign the document. Informed consent is not a contract, and the participant may withdraw from the trial at any time.

Institutional review board (IRB)   A committee of physicians, statisticians, researchers, community advocates, and others that ensures that a clinical trial is ethical and that the rights of study participants are protected. All clinical trials in the United Sates must be approved by an IRB before they begin. Every institution that conducts or supports biomedical or behavioral research involving human participants must, by federal regulation, have an IRB that initially approves and periodically reviews the research in order to protect the rights of human participants.

Intent to treat analysis   Analysis of clinical trial results that includes all data from participants in the groups to which they were randomized even if they never received the treatment.

Interventions   Primary interventions being studied.

Interim analysis   Analysis comparing intervention groups at any time before the formal completion of a trial, usually before recruitment is complete. Often used with stopping rules so that a trial can be stopped if participants are being put at risk unnecessarily. Timing and frequency of interim analyses should be specified in the protocol.

Investigational new drug (IND) A new drug, antibiotic drug or biological drug, that is used in a clinical investigation. It also includes a biological product used in vitro for diagnostic purposes.

Logarithmic scale A scale in which the logarithm of a value is used instead of the value. In a logarithmic scale on a RevMan forest plot, the distance between 1 and 10 is the same as the distance between 10 and 100, or between 100 and 1000. A logarithmic scale may be used when the range of numbers being represented is large, or to represent ratios. See also linear scale.

Logistic regression A form of regression analysis that models an individual's odds of disease or some other outcome as a function of a risk factor or intervention. It is widely used for dichotomous outcomes, in particular, to carry out adjusted analysis.

Masked Knowledge of the intervention assignment.

Medical device An intervention defined as:

- Used for diagnosis, cure, mitigation, treatment or prevention of a disease or condition
- Affects the structure and function of the body
- Does not achieve intended use through chemical reaction
- Is not metabolized

Mean An average value calculated by adding all the observations and dividing by the number of observations.

Mean difference (in meta-analysis) A method used to combine measures on continuous scales (e.g., weight), where the mean, standard deviation and sample size in each group is known. The weight given to the difference in means from each study (e.g., how much influence each study has on the overall results of the meta-analysis) is determined by the precision of its estimate of effect.

Median The value of the observation that comes half way when the observations are ranked in order.

Meta-analysis The use of statistical techniques in a systematic review to integrate the results of included studies. Sometimes misused as a synonym for systematic reviews, where the review includes a meta-analysis.

Multivariate analysis Measuring the impact of more than one variable at a time while analyzing a set of data, such as looking at the impact of age, sex, and occupation on a particular outcome. Performed using regression analysis.

Natural history study Study of the natural development of something (such as an organism or a disease) over a period of time.

New drug application (NDA)   An application submitted by the manufacturer of a drug to the FDA—after clinical trials have been completed—for a license to market the drug for a specified indication.

Normal distribution   A statistical distribution with known properties commonly used as the basis of models to analyze continuous data. Key assumptions in such analyses are that the data are symmetrically distributed about a mean value, and the shape of the distribution can be described using the mean and standard deviation.

Noninferiority trial   A trial designed to determine whether the effect of a new treatment is not worse than a standard treatment by more than a prespecified amount. A one-sided version of an equivalence trial.

Null hypothesis   The statistical hypothesis that one variable (e.g., which treatment a study participant was allocated to receive) has no association with another variable or set of variables (e.g., whether or not a study participant died), or that two or more population distributions do not differ from one another. In simplest terms, the null hypothesis states that the factor of interest (e.g., treatment) has no impact on outcome (e.g., risk of death).

Off-label use   A drug prescribed for conditions other than those approved by the FDA.

Open-label trial   A clinical trial in which doctors and participants know which drug or vaccine is being administered.

Orphan drugs   An FDA category that refers to medications used to treat diseases and conditions that occur rarely.

Observational study   A study in which the investigators do not seek to intervene, and simply observe the course of events. Changes or differences in one characteristic (e.g., whether or not people received the intervention of interest) are studied in relation to changes or differences in other characteristic(s).

Odds ratio   The ratio of the odds of an event in one group to the odds of an event in another group. In studies of treatment effect, the odds in the treatment group are usually divided by the odds in the control group. An odds ratio of one indicates no difference between comparison groups. For undesirable outcomes an OR that is less than one indicates that the intervention was effective in reducing the risk of that outcome. When the risk is small, odds ratios are very similar to risk ratios.

One-tailed test   A hypothesis test in which the values for which we can reject the null hypothesis are located entirely in one tail of the probability distribution. Testing whether one treatment is better than another (rather than testing whether one treatment is either better or worse than another) would be a one-tailed test. (Also called one-sided test.)

Open clinical trial   There are several possible meanings for this term:
1. A clinical trial in which the investigator and participant are aware which intervention is being used for which participant (i.e., not blinded). Random allocation may or may not be used in such trials. Sometimes called an "open label" design.
2. A clinical trial in which the investigator decides which intervention is to be used (nonrandom allocation). This is sometimes called an open label design (but some trials said to be "open label" are randomized).

Parallel group trial   A trial that compares two groups of people concurrently, one of which receives the intervention of interest and one of which is a control group. Some parallel trials have more than two comparison groups and some compare different interventions without including a nonintervention control group.

Per-protocol analysis   An analysis of the subset of participants from a randomized controlled trial who complied with the protocol sufficiently to ensure that their data would be likely to exhibit the effect of treatment. This subset may be defined after considering exposure to treatment, availability of measurements, and absence of major protocol deviations. The per-protocol analysis strategy may be subject to bias as the reasons for noncompliance may be related to treatment.

Posterior distribution   The outcome of Bayesian statistical analysis. A probability distribution describing how likely are different values of an outcome (e.g., treatment effect). It takes into account the belief before the study (the prior distribution) and the observed data from the study.

Prospective study   In evaluations of the effects of interventions, a study in which people are identified according to current risk status or exposure, and followed forward through time to observe outcome. Randomized controlled trials are always prospective studies. Cohort studies are commonly either prospective or retrospective, whereas case-control studies are usually retrospective. In Epidemiology, "prospective study" is sometimes misused as a synonym for cohort study.

P-value   The probability (ranging from zero to one) that the results observed in a study (or results more extreme) could have occurred by chance if in reality the null hypothesis was true. In a meta-analysis, the P-value for the overall effect assesses the overall statistical significance of the difference between the intervention groups, while the P-value for the heterogeneity statistic assesses the statistical significance of differences between the effects observed in each study.

Pharmacokinetics The processes (in a living organism) of absorption, distribution, metabolism, and excretion of a drug or vaccine.

Placebo A placebo is an inactive pill, liquid, or powder that has no treatment value. In clinical trials, experimental treatments are often compared with placebos to assess the treatment's effectiveness.

Placebo-controlled study A method of investigation of drugs in which an inactive substance (the placebo) is given to one group of participants while the drug being tested is given to another group.

Placebo effect A physical or emotional change, occurring after a substance is taken or administered, that is not the result of any special property of the substance. The change may be beneficial, reflecting the expectations of the participant and, often, the expectations of the person giving the substance.

Preclinical The testing of experimental therapies in the test tube or in animals—the testing that occurs before trials in humans may be carried out.

Prevention trials Trials to find better ways to prevent disease in people who have never had the disease or to prevent a disease from returning. These approaches may include medicines, vitamins, vaccines, minerals, or lifestyle changes.

Protocol A study plan on which all clinical trials are based. The plan is carefully designed to safeguard the health of the participants as well as answer specific research questions. A protocol describes what types of people may participate in the trial; the schedule of tests, procedures, medications, and dosages; and the length of the study. While in a clinical trial, participants following a protocol are seen regularly by the research staff to monitor their health and to determine the safety and effectiveness of their treatment.

Quality of life trials (or supportive care trials) Trials that explore ways to improve comfort and quality of life for individuals with a chronic illness.

Randomization A method based on chance by which study participants are assigned to a treatment group. Randomization minimizes the differences among groups by equally distributing people with particular characteristics among all the trial arms. The researchers do not know which treatment is better.

Randomized trial   A study in which participants are randomly (i.e., by chance) assigned to one of two or more treatment arms of a clinical trial. Occasionally placebos are utilized.

Side effects   Any undesired actions or effects of a drug or treatment. Experimental drugs must be evaluated for both immediate and long-term side effects.

Single-blind study   A study in which one party, either the investigator or participant, is unaware of what medication the participant is taking.

Standard treatment   A treatment currently in wide use and approved by the FDA, considered to be effective in the treatment of a specific disease or condition.

Standards of care   Treatment regimen or medical management based on state of the art participant care.

Statistical significance   The probability that an event or difference occurred by chance alone.

Study endpoint   A primary or secondary outcome used to judge the effectiveness of a treatment.

Sensitivity analysis   An analysis used to determine how sensitive the results of a study or systematic review are to changes in how it was done. Sensitivity analyses are used to assess how robust the results are in correlation to uncertain decisions or assumptions about the data and the methods that were used.

Standard deviation (SD)   A measure of the spread or dispersion of a set of observations, calculated as the average difference from the mean value in the sample.

Standard error (SE)   The standard deviation of the sampling distribution of a statistic. Measurements taken from a sample of the population will vary from sample to sample. The standard error is a measure of the variation in the sample statistic over all possible samples of the same size. The standard error decreases as the sample size increases.

Statistically significant   A result that is unlikely to have happened by chance. The usual threshold for this judgment is that the results, or more extreme results, would occur by chance with a probability of less than 0.05 if the null hypothesis was true. Statistical tests produce a *P*-value to assess this.

Stratification   The process by which groups are separated into mutually exclusive subgroups of the population that share a characteristic, such as age group, sex, or socioeconomic status. It is possible to compare these different strata to try and see if the effects of a treatment differ between the subgroups. See also subgroup analysis.

Stopping rule   A procedure that allows interim analyses in clinical trials at predefined times, while preserving the type I error at some prespecified level.

Subgroup analysis   An analysis in which the intervention effect is evaluated in a defined subset of the participants in a trial, or in complementary subsets, such as by sex or in age categories. Trial sizes are generally too small for subgroup analyses to have adequate statistical power.

Surrogate endpoints   Often physiological or biochemical markers that can be relatively quickly and easily measured, and that are taken as being predictive of important clinical outcomes. They are often used when observation of clinical outcomes requires long follow-up. For example, blood pressure is not directly important to patients, but it is often used as an outcome in clinical trials because it is a risk factor for stroke and heart attacks.

Retrospective study   A study in which the outcomes have occurred to the participants before the study commenced. Case-control studies are usually retrospective, cohort studies sometimes are, and randomized controlled trials never are.

***t*-Test**   A statistical hypothesis test derived from the *t* distribution. It is used to compare continuous data in two groups (also called Student's *t*-test).

Toxicity   An adverse effect produced by a drug that is detrimental to the participant's health. The level of toxicity associated with a drug will vary, depending on the condition that the drug is used to treat.

Two-tailed *t*-test   A hypothesis test in which the values for which we can reject the null hypothesis are located entirely in both tails of the probability distribution. Testing whether one treatment is better or worse than another (rather than testing whether one treatment is only better than another) would be a two-tailed test (also called two-sided test).

Washout period/phase   In a cross-over trial, the stage after the first treatment is withdrawn, but before the second treatment is started. The washout period aims to allow time for any active effects of the first treatment to wear off before the new one gets started.

REFERENCES

1. Franciosi LG, Butterfield NN, MacLeod BA. Evaluating the process of generating a clinical trial protocol. *Proc AMIA* 2002:1021.
2. Chiacchlerini RP. Medical device clinical trial design, conduct, and analysis. In: *Health Care Technology Policy I: The Role of Technology in the Cost of Health Care* 1994:278–85.
3. Smith-Tyler J. Informed consent, confidentiality, and subject rights in clinical trials. *Proc Am Thorac Soc* 2007;4(2):189–93.
4. Schweickert W, Hall J. Informed consent in the intensive care unit: ensuring understanding in a complex environment. *Curr Opin Crit Care* 2005;11(6):624–8.
5. Gammelgaard A. Informed consent in acute myocardial infarction research. *J Med Philos* 2004;29(4):417–34.
6. Morin K, Rakatansky H, Riddick FA Jr, Morse LJ, O'Bannon JM 3rd, Goldrich MS, Ray P, Weiss M, Sade RM, Spillman MA. Managing conflicts of interest in the conduct of clinical trials. *JAMA* 2002;287(1):78–84.
7. Helft PR, Ratain MJ, Epstein RA, Siegler M. Inside information: financial conflicts of interest for research subjects in early phase clinical trials. *J Natl Cancer Inst* 2004;96(9):656–61.
8. Sandman L, Mosher A, Khan A, Tapy J, Condos R, Ferrell S, Vernon A, Tuberculosis Trials Consortium. Quality assurance in a large clinical trials consortium: the experience of the Tuberculosis Trials Consortium. *Contemp Clin Trials* 2006;27(6):554–60.

9. Leap LL. Reporting of adverse events. *NEJM* 2002;347:1633–8.

10. Rogers AS, Israel E, Smith CR. Physician knowledge, attitudes, and behavior related to reporting adverse drug events. *Arch Intern Med* 1988;148:1589–92.

11. DeMets D, Califf R, Dixon D, Ellenberg S, Fleming T, Held P, Julian D, Kaplan R, Levine R, Neaton J, Packer M, Pocock S, Rockhold F, Seto B, Siegel J, Snapinn S, Stump D, Temple R, Whitley R. Issues in regulatory guidelines for data monitoring committees. *Clin Trials* 2004;1(2): 162–9.

12. Morse MA, Califf RM, Sugarman J. Monitoring and ensuring safety during clinical research. *JAMA* 2001;285:1201–5.

13. Lindquist M, Edwards IR. The WHO Programme for International Drug Monitoring, its database, and the technical support of the Uppsala Monitoring Center. *J Rheumatol* 2001;28:1180–7.

14. Kessler DA. Introducing MEDWatch. A new approach to reporting medication and device adverse effects and product problems. *JAMA* 1993;269(21):2765–8.

15. Wittes J, Lakatos E, Probstfield J. Surrogate endpoints in clinical trials: cardiovascular diseases. *Stat Med* 1989;8(4):415–25.

16. Prentice RL. Surrogate endpoints in clinical trials: Definition and operational criteria. *Stat Med* 1989;8(4):431–40.

17. Gordon DJ. Cholesterol lowering and total mortality. In: Rifkind BM, ed. *Contemporary Issues in Cholesterol Lowering: Clinical and Population Aspects*. New York: Marcel Dekker; 1994.

18. Collins R, Peto R, MacMahon S, Hebert P, Fiebach NH, Eberlein KA, et al. Blood pressure, stroke, and coronary heart disease. Part 2, Short-term reductions in blood pressure: overview of randomized drug trials in their epidemiological context. *Lancet* 1990;335:827–38.

19. Kleist P. Composite endpoints for clinical trials: current perspectives. *Int J Pharmaceut Med* 2007;21(3):187–98.

20. The CAPRICORN Investigators. Effect of Carvedilol on outcome after myocardial Infarction in patients with left-ventricular dysfunction: the CAPRICORN randomised trial. *Lancet* 2001;357:1385–90.

21. Blackwelder WC. "Proving the null hypothesis" in clinical trials. *Control Clin Trials* 1982;3:345–52.

22. Donner A. Approaches to sample size estimation in the design of clinical trials. *Stat Med* 1984;3:199–214.

23. Wittes J. Sample size calculations for randomized controlled trials. *Epidemiol Rev* 2002;24:39–53.

24. Altman DG. Confidence intervals for the number needed to treat. *BMJ* 1998;317:1309–12.

25. Briggs A. Economic evaluation and clinical trials: size matters: the need for greater power in cost analyses poses an ethical dilemma. *BMJ* 2000;321(7273):1362–3.

26. Bernardo JM, Smith AF. *Bayesian Statistical Theory*. New York: Wiley, 2000.

27. French S, Smith JQ, eds. *The Practice of Bayesian Analysis*. New York: Wiley, 1997.

28. Geller J. FDA issues new guidance on device clinical trials and lessens the burden on IVD makers. *J Clin Eng* 2006;31(3):119–20.

29. Fleiss JL. The statistical basis of meta-analysis. *Stat Meth Med Res* 1993;2: 121–45.

30. Higgins PT, Thompson SG, Deeks JJ, Altman DG. Measuring inconsistency in meta-analysis. *BMJ* 2003;327:557–60.

31. Normand SLT. Meta-analysis: formulating, evaluating, combining and reporting. *Stat Med* 1999;18:321–59.

32. Whitehead A. *Meta-analysis of controlled clinical trials*. New York: Wiley, 2002.

33. Pocock SJ, Clayton TC, Altman DG. Survival plots of time-to-event outcomes in clinical trials: good practice and pitfalls. *Lancet* 2002;359: 1686–9.

34. Newell DJ. Intention-to-treat analysis: implications for quantitative and qualitative research. *Int J Epidemiol* 1992;21:837–41.

35. Bulpitt C. *Randomised Controlled Clinical Trials*, 2nd ed. Dordreicht: Kluwer Academic.

36. Auleley GR, Giraudeau B, Baron G, Maillefert JF, Dougados M, Ravaud P. The methods for handling missing data in clinical trials influence sample size requirements. *J Clin Epidemiol* 2004;57(5):447–53.

37. Scott PE, Campbell G. Interpretation of subgroup analyses in medical device clinical trials. *Drug Inf J* 1997;32:213–20.

38. Warda HM, Warda H, Bax J, Bosch J, Atsma D, Jukemi J, Van der Wall E, Schalij M, Demrawsingh P. Effect of intracoronary aqueous oxygen on left ventricular remodeling after anterior wall ST-elevation acute myocardial infarction. *Am J Cardiol* 2005;96(1):22–4.

39. Chatfield C, Collins AJ. *Introduction to Multivariate Analysis*. Oxford, UK: Chapman and Hall/CRC, 1981.

40. Emanuel EJ, Wendler D, Grady C. What makes clinical research ethical? *JAMA* 2000;283(20):2701–11.

41. Ellenberg S, Fleming T. *Data Monitoring Committees in Clinical Trials: A Practical Perspective*. New York: Wiley, 2002.

42. Dickersin K, Rennie D. Registering clinical trials. *JAMA* 2003;290(4): 516–23.

43. FDA guidance document for ClinTrials.gov (http://www.fda.gov/cder/guidance/4856fnl.htm).

44. Chow SC, Liu JP. *Design and Analysis of Clinical Trials: Concept and Methodologies*. New York: Wiley, 1998.

45. Friedman LM, Furberg CD, Demets D. *Fundamentals of Clinical Trials*, 3rd ed. New York: Springer Verlag, 1998.

46. Fleiss JL. *Design and Analysis of Clinical Experiments*. New York: John Wiley, 1986.

47. Pocock SJ. *Clinical Trials: A Practical Approach*. New York: Wiley, 1983.

48. Cox DR. Regression models and life tables. *J Roy Stat Soc* 1972;B34:187–220. Cochran WG, Cox GM. *Experimental Design*, 2nd ed. New York: Wiley, 1957.

49. Mulrow CD, Cook DJ, Davidoff F. Systematic reviews: critical links in the great chain of evidence. *Ann Intern Med* 1997;126(5):389–91.

50. Senn S. *Cross-over Trials in Clinical Research*, 2nd ed. New York: Wiley, 2002.

51. Lao CS. Application and analysis of repeated-measure design in medical device clinical trials: statistical considerations. *J Biopharm Stat* 2000;10(3):433–45.

52. Gayet JL. The OPTIMAAL trial: losartan or captopril after acute myocardial infarction. *Lancet* 2002;360:1884–5.

53. Hill RA, Dündar Y, Bakhai A, Dickson R, Walley T. Drug-eluting stents: an early systematic review to inform policy. *Eur Heart J* 2004;25:902–19.

54. Chen E, Sapirstein W, Ahn C, Swain J, Zuckerman B. FDA perspective on clinical trial design for cardiovascular devices. *Ann Thorac Surg* 2006;82(3):773–5.

55. Parides MK, Moskowitz AJ, Ascheim DD, Rose EA, Gelijns AC. Progress versus precision: challenges in clinical trial design for left ventricular assist devices. *Ann Thorac Surg* 2006;82(3):1140–6.

56. Grunkemeier GL, Jin R, Starr A. Prosthetic heart valves: objective performance criteria versus randomized clinical trial. *Ann Thorac Surg* 2006;82(3):776–80.

57. Zuckerman BD, Muni NI. Cardiovascular device development: an FDA perspective. *Am J Ther* 2005;12(2):176–8.

58. http://www.accessdata.fda.gov/scripts/cdrh/cfadvisory/details.cfm?mtg=266.

59. Transatlantic inter-society consensus (TASC) on management of peripheral arterial disease (PAD). *J Vasc Surg* 2000;31:1–296.

60. ICAI Study Group. Prostanoids for chronic critical leg ischemia: a randomized, controlled, open-label trial with Prostaglandin E1. *Ann Intern Med* 1999;130:412–21.

61. FDA Summary of Safety and Effectiveness (P040012). ACCULINK carotid stent system and RX ACCULINK carotid stent system, 2004.

62. North American Symptomatic Carotid Endarterectomy Trial. Methods, patient characteristics, and progress. *Stroke* 1991;22(6):711–20.

63. Barnett HJ, Taylor DW, Eliasziw M, Fox AJ, Ferguson GG, Haynes RB, Rankin RN, Clagett GP, Hachinski VC, Sackett DL, Thorpe KE, Meldrum HE. Benefit of carotid endarterectomy in patients with symptomatic moderate or severe stenosis. North American Symptomatic Carotid Endarterectomy Trial Collaborators. *N Engl J Med* 1998;339(20):1415–25.

64. Endarterectomy for asymptomatic carotid artery stenosis. Executive Committee for the Asymptomatic Carotid Atherosclerosis Study. *JAMA* 1995;273(18):1421–8.

65. Department of Health and Human Services, Office of Inspector General. The globalization of clinical trials: a growing challenge in protecting human subjects. September 2001 OEI-01-00-00190. http://oig.hhs.gov/oei.

66. Macrae DJ. The Council for International Organizations and Medical Sciences (CIOMS) guidelines on ethics of clinical trials. *Proc Am Thorac Soc* 2007;4(2):176–8.

67. Dreyfuss D. Beyond randomized, controlled trials. *Curr Opin Crit Care* 2004;10(6):574–8.

INDEX

Design, Execution, and Management of Medical Device Clinical Trials,
by Salah Abdel-aleem
Copyright © 2009 John Wiley & Sons, Inc.

Printed and bound by CPI Group (UK) Ltd, Croydon, CR0 4YY

16/04/2025

14658523-0004